W9-AMV-926

Olaf College

JAN 5 1983

Science Library

UNDERSTANDING
IMMUNOLOGY

UNDERSTANDING IMMUNOLOGY

Alastair J. Cunningham

Department of Microbiology
John Curtin School of Medical Research
Canberra City, Australia

ACADEMIC PRESS   New York   San Francisco   London
A Subsidiary of Harcourt Brace Jovanovich, Publishers

QR
181
C78

COPYRIGHT © 1978, BY ACADEMIC PRESS, INC.
ALL RIGHTS RESERVED.
NO PART OF THIS PUBLICATION MAY BE REPRODUCED OR
TRANSMITTED IN ANY FORM OR BY ANY MEANS, ELECTRONIC
OR MECHANICAL, INCLUDING PHOTOCOPY, RECORDING, OR ANY
INFORMATION STORAGE AND RETRIEVAL SYSTEM, WITHOUT
PERMISSION IN WRITING FROM THE PUBLISHER.

ACADEMIC PRESS, INC.
111 Fifth Avenue, New York, New York 10003

United Kingdom Edition published by
ACADEMIC PRESS, INC. (LONDON) LTD.
24/28 Oval Road, London NW1

Library of Congress Cataloging in Publication Data

Cunningham, Alastair J
    Understanding immunology.

    Includes bibliographies and index.
    1.   Immunology.   I.   Title.   [DNLM: 1.   Immunity.
QW504 O73u]
QR181.C78   616.07'9   77-24680
ISBN 0−12−199870−3 (cloth)
ISBN 0−12−199872−X (paper)

PRINTED IN THE UNITED STATES OF AMERICA
79 80 81 82   9 8 7 6 5 4 3

TO MY MOTHER

Contents

4   Lymphocytes, Lymphoid Tissue, and Antibody Forming Cells

5   Immunocompetent Cells and Induction of the Antibody Response

6   Memory and Tolerance

Preface

Immunology is an intensely interesting field, but is one that can be confusing to the newcomer. The subject began as a study of immunity to infectious disease, and broadened enormously to encompass aspects of many other biological topics such as genetics, transplantation, cancer, and cell differentiation. The phenomena now included in immunology are numerous and complex. The jargon has become formidable enough to deter many nonspecialists. Yet modern immunology is sufficiently advanced to display clearly a number of simple, unifying principles that, once grasped, form a background against which most observations can be rationally explained. This book is an attempt to describe the subject in a logical manner by emphasizing these principles.

The point of view taken is one with which most immunologists would agree: that the immune system has evolved to combat infectious disease. It is a system that adapts to the environment, operating through a population of lymphoid cells among which variants appear and are selected by antigens. There is a constant need to avoid reactions against self. The way in which the immune system manages to react against virtually any foreign substance but not against its "host" is seen as the central problem in the discipline. The many controversial areas in immunology have not been avoided. On the contrary, they have been thoroughly "aired" in order to bring the reader to a point where he can experience vicariously some of the excitement of current research. I have, in general, expressed my own opinions, but have cautioned the reader against accepting them uncritically.

The book is based on a series of lectures presented to science undergraduates at the Australian National University. It is hoped that it will prove useful as an introduction to immunology to those with some background in biology: undergraduate or graduate students as well as established researchers in other fields. For those interested in greater detail, the literature can be researched using the books and reviews referred to at the end of each chapter. The questions and answers also appended to each chapter should improve the usefulness of the text as a basis for a lecture course in immunology.

I would like to acknowledge invaluable training in the laboratories of Drs. W. A. Te Punga, S. Fazekas de St. Groth, K. J. Lafferty, G. J. V. Nossal, N. A.

Mitchison, L. A. Herzenberg, and G. L. Ada, and to admit to the strong influence of the writings of F. M. Burnet, N. K. Jerne, M. Cohn, and P. A. Bretscher. Many colleagues criticized chapters of the manuscript, and the following people kindly read large parts of it: Gordon Ada, Jim Arnold, Bob Blandon, Vivienne Bracciale, Tom Bracciale, Peter Bretscher, Don Capra, Marion Cunningham, Dave Jackson, Maurice Landy, Richard Pink, Ian Ramshaw, Pam Russell, and Ted Steele. I am particularly grateful to Lesley Russell for her critical review of the entire manuscript and for other advice, and to my wife Margaret for patiently typing it all.

Alastair J. Cunningham*

*Present address: Department of Medical Biophysics, Ontario Cancer Institute, Toronto, Ontario, Canada.

Basic Requirements and Properties of an Immune System

Where is the knowledge we have lost in information?

T. S. Eliot

Living things have a precarious existence. They are constantly threatened by changes in their environment, such as alterations in climate or competition by new kinds of neighbors, and changes like these have eliminated many species. Fortunately, the new conditions usually develop over many generations, allowing time for evolutionary adaptation by mutation and selection of offspring better suited than their ancestors to the new surroundings.

There is also, in the environment of any species, another important type of potentially harmful change which is much more rapid: the onset of infectious disease. A vertebrate is an attractive culture medium for many kinds of viral, bacterial, fungal, and metazoan parasites. Viruses and bacteria, in particular, with their capacity for extremely rapid multiplication, may cause an epidemic which sweeps through a population within weeks. Against such rapid change, the evolution of new and resistant offspring within a slow-breeding vertebrate species is a relatively inefficient defense. Vertebrates have had to develop a way by which the *individual* may protect itself against invasion: this is the immune response,* a reaction by the animal, aimed at neutralizing or removing infectious organisms or foreign bodies.

It should gradually become clear, as we progress through this book, that the very successful principles of variation and natural selection have been used within the body to provide this immune response. The response is mediated by a population of free-floating individual cells among which variants appear and are

---

*An alternative view of the evolutionary pressures favoring development of the immune response is discussed in Chapter 14, while in Chapter 15 we will examine some possible reasons for the ability of invertebrates and plants to manage without any adaptive immunity.

selected, the whole process occurring within a time scale of days or weeks rather than thousands of years.

1.1 THE BASIC PATTERN OF AN IMMUNE RESPONSE

When a foreign substance or *antigen* (e.g., a population of bacteria) gains entry into an animal, *antibodies* to that antigen may appear in the serum. These antibodies are molecules which can react with the antigen in various detectable ways; their amount varies with time after injection, as shown in Fig. 1.1. We will discuss such responses and define terms more fully in subsequent chapters, but for the present we should note four main features:

a. An immune response is *specific,* that is, antibodies are produced which react with the injected antigen but not usually with other foreign substances.

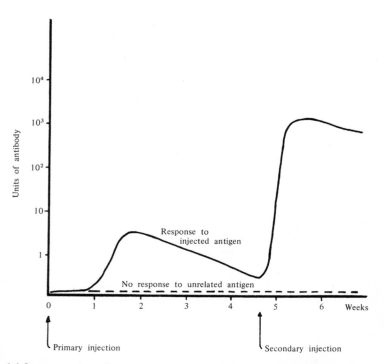

Fig. 1.1 Immune response by an animal injected with two doses of the same antigen, 4 weeks apart. Serum antibody levels have been measured. Such responses vary greatly with the species and antigens used.

b. A vast number of different antibodies to different antigens is possible; that is, the response is potentially *diverse*.

c. It is *adaptive*, that is, the strength and nature of the immune reaction changes with time after antigenic stimulation. Figure 1.1 shows how the amount of specific antibody in serum rises after first exposure to antigen. A second injection usually provokes a more rapid and greater rise in antibody, indicating that the animal "remembered" its first contact with that antigen (see Chapter 6).

d. Finally, responses may be induced even by what seem to be *unexpected* antigens, that is, antigens not previously encountered by the species, such as new microorganisms or synthetic compounds.

Let us now try to find some of the reasons why the immune response shows these four properties.

1.2 BASIC REQUIREMENTS OF AN IMMUNE SYSTEM

1.2.1 Specificity

There is an enormous variety of foreign substances against which the immune system may be called upon to react (Fig. 1.2). A reasonable question might be: "Why not have one or a few superantibodies, each able to deal with many different infectious organisms or other foreign bodies?" The problem is that such superantibodies would certainly react against intrinsic components of the animal. The host animal which is making the antibody is itself very complex and contains many thousands of different types of molecules, some of which resemble foreign antigens. We would expect that the more versatile the antibody, i.e., the more foreign particles or antigens which it could recognize, the more danger there would be that it would also react with a self-component. Conversely, a highly specific antibody able to recognize only one antigen would run less risk of also recognizing and perhaps reacting in a harmful way with one of the host's own self-components. It was Paul Ehrlich (see Table 1.1) who realized that animals must not make antibodies against parts of themselves. This requirement forces antibodies to be specific. The immune response is a constant search for molecules which react with foreign antigens but not with one's self. How this is achieved is the central problem in immunology.

1.2.2 Diversity

The next property follows directly from this need for specificity in immune responses. There are large numbers of different foreign antigens, against almost any of which antibody can be produced. There are also thousands of self-

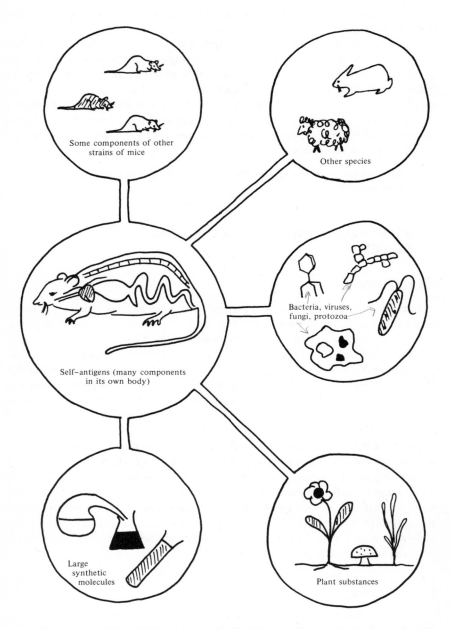

Fig. 1.2 The antigenic universe (from the point of view of an experimental mouse).

TABLE 1.1
History of Ideas in Immunology[a]

	Cells	Antibodies and immunity	Ideas on generation of diversity and self-tolerance
Ancient times		Recovery → Immunity	
1800		Jenner: vaccination against cowpox protects against smallpox	
1880		Pasteur: attenuation of organisms to make vaccines	
1890	Metchnikoff: phagocytosis Denys and Leclef: phagocytosis enhanced by immunization	Rational basis for vaccination Von Behring: antibodies in serum Buchner, Bordet: complement	Ehrlich: side chain selective theory
1900	Wright: opsonins in phagocytosis	Landsteiner: blood groups and natural isohemagglutinins Ehrlich: quantitative measures of antigen–antibody combination Portier and Richet: immediate hypersensitivity	
1920	Zinsser: distinguished immediate and delayed hypersensitivity		
1930		Landsteiner: antibody specificity Heidelberger and Kendall: quantitative precipitation of antigen and antibody	Haurowitz, Mudd, and Alexander: instructive theory
1940	Chase: transfer of delayed hypersensitivity with cells Fagreus: nature of antibody-forming cells		Burnet and Fenner: self-tolerance
1950	Coons: detecting antibody-forming cells	Porter; Edelman: antibody structure	Billingham, Brent, and Medawar: self-tolerance by grafting cells Jerne; Talmage; Burnet: selective theories
1960	Nossal: 1 cell → 1 antibody Gowans: small lymphocytes as precursor cells Claman; Davies; Miller; Mitchison: cell cooperation for induction		
1970			Suppressor cells in tolerance; rapid clonal variation after antigen; network theory

[a] For more details see the entertaining introduction to the textbook by Humphrey and White (Ref. 1.3).

components which must be left alone. The only safe way to ensure this seems to be to have many different antibodies, each able to recognize, or react specifically, with a very limited range of molecular structures. After somehow removing antibodies which happen to react with self, we are still left with a sufficient variety to deal with foreign substances, providing that these are at least partly different in structure from self-components.

1.2.3 Adaptivity

We can see that a system capable of specifically reacting with an almost unlimited number of molecular shapes must have many different recognizing components. It follows that any one component will only be a small part of the whole. The amount of one particular antibody may need to be amplified greatly before there will be enough of it to have a useful effect, such as the elimination of infecting organisms as quickly as possible. The immune system therefore has to be *adaptive*. It first makes a large number of antibodies which are useful in counteracting a particular infection, and then, as we will see, a "memory" of this process is imprinted on the system so that in the event of reinfection by the same organism, a second reaction can be more rapid.

1.2.4 The Ability to Respond to Unexpected Stimuli

The three properties of specificity, diversity, and adaptivity are important for the immune system but are by no means unique to it—all may be found among enzymes and hormones, for example. There is, however, a further characteristic which is crucial, and highly developed only in immune and nervous systems: the ability to respond to *unexpected** stimuli. The enormous variety of possible antigens makes it probable that individuals will encounter some which were never before experienced by the species. In particular, this is true of infectious organisms. There are thousands of potentially dangerous kinds, and new variants arise rapidly, as the pathogens, which also seek to survive, produce offspring which are resistant to the defenses of their hosts. It is likely that an animal with a fixed "repertoire" of possible responses, even a very large repertoire, would eventually succumb to a variant against which it had no effective immunity. We can understand why the immune system has had to evolve as a flexible device capable of learning from the environment. An analogy may be drawn with the brain, which is also a learning device whose specific abilities depend on the environment it encounters: any of us can learn an entirely new language, for example.

This can be contrasted with all other "systems," e.g., the digestive processes. The gastrointestinal tract knows what to expect. It will break down only certain

---

*This fundamental property has been discussed by Mel Cohn in a brilliant essay (see Ref. 1.7).

kinds of foods and needs a limited number of "responses," in this case, digestive enzymes. For a species to "learn" to make a new enzyme capable of utilizing a new substrate, many thousands of years of evolution would be required.

1.3 SUMMARY

The immune system has four main properties:

1. Like the nervous system, but unlike most others, it has the capacity to respond to *unexpected* stimuli, stimuli which were not a regular part of the environment of the evolving species.

2. The immune response has to be *specific,* so as to react against foreign substances but not self-components.

3. The need for specific reactivity to a great variety of foreign bodies or antigens means that the immune system is *diverse:* it has many different effector molecules.

4. A response involves selecting a suitable specific effector molecule, initially present in small amounts among many others, and amplifying this to useful levels, that is, the response is *adaptive.*

FURTHER READING

1.1   Burnet, F. M. (1969). "Cellular Immunology," Books 1 and 2. Melbourne University Press, Melbourne.
1.2   Hobart, M. J. and McConnell, I. (1975). "The Immune System." Blackwell Scientific Publ., Oxford.
1.3   Humphrey, J. H. and White R. G. (1970). "Immunology for Students of Medicine," 3rd ed. Blackwell Scientific Publ., Oxford.
1.4   Nossal, G. J. V. (1971). "Antibodies and Immunity." Pelican. An excellent account for the nonscientific reader.
1.5   Roitt, I. M. (1974). "Essential Immunology," 2nd ed. Blackwell Scientific Publ., Oxford.
1.6   Rose, N. R., Milgrom, F., and van Oss (eds.). (1973). "Principles of Immunology." Macmillan, New York.
1.7   Cohn, M. (1968). Molecular biology of expectation. *In* "Nucleic Acids in Immunology" (O. J. Plescia and W. Brown, eds.), p. 671. Springer-Verlag, New York. Discusses the ability of the immune system to respond to unexpected stimuli. Cohn's papers are too difficult for most beginners, but will amply repay study by more advanced readers.
1.8   Cohn, M. (1972). "Immunology: What Are the Rules of the Game?" *Cell. Immunol.* **5,** 1.

MAJOR JOURNALS

Aust. J. Exp. Biol. Med. Sci.; Cell. Immunol.; Clin. Exp. Immunol.; Eur. J. Immunol.; Immunochemistry; Immunology; Int. Arch. Allergy Appl. Immunol.; J. Exp. Med.; J. Immunogenet.; J. Immunol.; J. Immunol. Methods; J. Reticuloendothel. Soc.; Lancet; Nature (London); Proc. Natl. Acad. Sci. (U.S.A.); Scand. J. Immunol. Science; Transplantation

PERIODICAL REVIEWS

Adv. Immunol., Academic Press, London; *Contemp. Top. Immunobiol.*, Plenum Press, New York; *Contemp. Top. Mol. Immunol.*, Plenum Press, New York; *Prog. Allergy*, S. Karger, Basel; *Prog. Immunol.* [Proceedings of International Immunology Congresses, held every 3 years, and a useful review of current knowledge in all branches of the subject. Number II, 1974, L. Brent and E. J. Holborow (eds.). North Holland, Amsterdam. Number III: Sydney, 1977]; *Transplant. Rev.* (G. Moller, ed.). Munksgaard, Copenhagen. (A particularly good series for the student of modern immunological ideas. Name changed in 1977 to *Immunol. Rev.*)

QUESTIONS

1.1   Human patients who receive an organ graft (e.g., a kidney) from another individual are routinely treated with *immunosuppressant* drugs. Such drugs depress immune responses generally. Why are they given, and what are their side effects likely to be?

1.2   What would happen to a helminth parasite which managed to acquire an outer "coat" of substances derived from its host?

1.3   We have mentioned that a second immune response to an antigen is often faster and stronger than the first response to the same antigen given some weeks or months earlier. This adaptivity has its negative aspect: sometimes prior exposure to an antigen will decrease a secondary reaction against that substance (immunological tolerance, Chapter 6). If an individual was injected with a foreign antigen in early fetal life and at regular intervals thereafter, what would you predict about the individual's immune responsiveness against that antigen later in life?

1.4   List some areas of human and veterinary clinical medicine where immunological phenomena are important.

1.5   Some individuals in a population of microorganisms commonly survive even when exposed to an entirely new, toxic drug (e.g., antibiotic). Why? If a human has roughly 10^{12} cells making up his immune system, will these all be genetically identical?

2

The Reaction of Antibody with Antigen

There is a circular definition at the heart of immunology. *Antigen* is whatever stimulates the production of antibody, and *antibodies* are molecules whose production is induced by antigen. Like many concepts in this discipline and in other branches of biology, the terms "antigen" and "antibody" are difficult to define in a simple way, but their meaning becomes clearer with time and thought. For the present, we can say that *antigens* are any substances which, when introduced into an animal, provoke a specific immune response. This response is often measured as antibody capable of reaction with the antigen, although other types of specific immune response (e.g., "cellular," Chapter 9) are also seen. Antigens may be particulate, e.g., bacteria, viruses, erythrocytes from other species, or soluble, e.g., proteins, polysaccharides, or combinations of proteins and polysaccharides together or with lipids. Nucleic acids and lipids by themselves are usually not antigenic. We apply the adjective "immune" equally to reactions against living or nonliving materials. Substances do not normally act as antigens unless they have a molecular weight of more than about 5,000–10,000 (the reasons for this will emerge later), and as a broad generalization, *immunogenicity,* or the ability of an antigen to stimulate a response, increases with molecular size. Particles such as bacteria, red blood cells, or aggregated proteins are often the strongest antigens. Substances derived from living organisms are usually only antigenic in different, and preferably genetically distant, species. A mouse will make antibody very well to sheep erythrocytes, rather poorly to rat erythrocytes, and usually not at all to its own erythrocytes. The immunogenicity of a molecule is not an absolute property but a relative one: it depends on the animal in which it is tested.

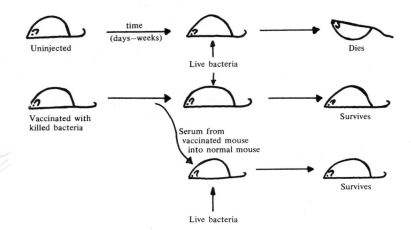

Fig. 2.1 <u>Acquired immunological resistance</u>. Model experiment demonstrating that mice previously injected with killed bacteria have become resistant to an inoculum of live bacteria which would prove fatal to normal mice. In some cases this immunity can be "passively" transferred by injecting serum from the immune animals into otherwise normal recipients.

2.1 MAIN PROPERTIES OF ANTIBODIES

Antibodies are the most important known effector molecules of the immune system. We can illustrate some of their properties by examining the experimental model shown in Fig. 2.1. If killed bacteria are injected into mice, these mice may, within days, become "immune" or resistant to a subsequent injection ("challenge") of live bacteria capable of killing normal, unimmunized animals. In investigating the reasons for this resistance we would notice several things:

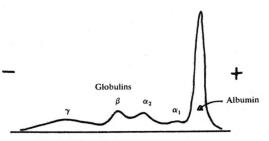

Fig. 2.2 Serum proteins. Separation of human serum globulins by electrophoresis on paper or cellulose acetate. When the bands are stained and scanned with a densitometer, the area under the peaks is proportional to the concentration of the component. Most antibody activity is found in the γ-globulin region, and some in the β-globulin.

(a) When the blood from an immune animal is mixed with the live bacteria it may kill them. We would find that the serum, the fluid fraction of blood left after clotting, had the same property as whole blood.

(b) Analyzing this further we might fractionate the serum by electrophoresis (Fig. 2.2) and test each fraction for activity. We would find the neutralizing or protective activity in the globulin region, particularly among the gamma-globulin, as was first demonstrated by Tiselius and Kabat, in 1937.

(c) If serum taken at different times was titrated, that is, if we determined how far it could be diluted before losing its neutralizing effect when mixed with a standard number of bacteria (Fig. 2.3), we would obtain a graph similar to that

1. Collect serum from animal immunized against a bacterial culture

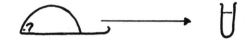

2. Make serial dilutions of this serum

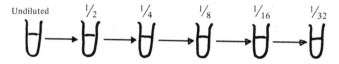

3. Add a standard number of bacteria to each tube, and mix. (Complement, Section 2.2.6, may also be needed to kill the bacteria.)

4. Standard volume from each tube plated out on agar growth medium

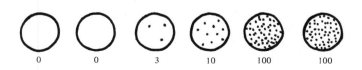

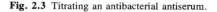

5. Number of colony–forming bacteria remaining indicates the point at which serum antibody activity was lost by dilution

Fig. 2.3 Titrating an antibacterial antiserum.

illustrated in Fig. 1.1. The potency or titer of a serum waxes and then wanes with time after antigenic stimulation.

(d) We would usually find little difference in the total amount of gamma-globulin in the serum of immune and normal mice, as opposed to the large increase (sometimes many thousandfold) in the specific killing power of immune serum. This tells us several things. First, the gamma-globulin molecules cannot all have identical structure, otherwise some correlation between total amount and neutralizing activity would be expected. Rather, there must be a minority population of molecules with the power to affect the immunizing bacteria. We could confirm this by absorbing the serum with bacteria, that is, by mixing the two and centrifuging out the bacteria with the specific antibody combined to them. The supernatant serum should now have lost its specific activity without losing more than a small proportion of its total gamma-globulins. Absorbing with an un-related bacterial species would have no effect. So the minority population, in-duced by the antigen, has the power to bind specifically to that antigen, but not to another.

(e) As an extra refinement, we might try injecting a mouse with two dif-ferent kinds of bacteria, after which it should become resistant to challenge (reinjection) with either. The serum would now contain antibody molecules able to kill either bacterium. Each type of activity could be separately and specifically removed from serum only by absorption with the corresponding bacterial type.

This model experiment, which is a composite of many routine immunological operations, has revealed several of the properties of antibodies. They are *im-munoglobulins*, proteins which appear in the globulin fraction of serum after an animal is stimulated with antigen, and they can combine with that antigen but not usually with others. Their detailed structure is discussed in the next chapter.

2.2 WAYS OF DETECTING ANTIBODY

Serum antibodies are "windows" through which the experimentalist or clini-cian may view the progress of an immune response. There are many ways of detecting them; much of the often complicated phenomenology of the subject involves ingenious assay systems for measuring antibody in serum (*serological tests*). We will now briefly discuss several of the more important techniques. (More details can be found in some of the texts referred to at the end of this chapter.)

2.2.1 Antigen Binding

The basic property of antibody is its power to bind to the antigen which induced it. Those assays for antibody activity which are simplest in principle use this property only: other tests (described below) require the antibody to do

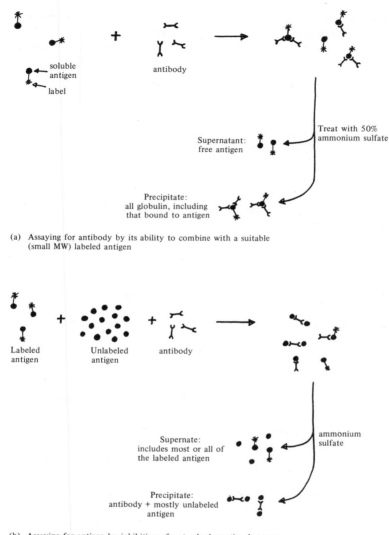

(a) Assaying for antibody by its ability to combine with a suitable (small MW) labeled antigen

(b) Assaying for antigen by inhibition of a standard reaction between antibody and labeled antigen

Fig. 2.4 Antigen-binding assays.

something else after initial binding. A simple binding assay may be set up by reacting a standard amount of radioactively labeled antigen with a test antiserum (Fig. 2.4). Antigen which has complexed with antibody can now be separated from free antigen in various ways. For example, if the antigen is soluble in 50% saturated ammonium sulfate solution, this high salt concentration may be used to precipitate all globulin in the mixture, including that bound to antigen. The amount of antigen bound provides a measure of the antibody *activity* in the serum. This kind of test has many variations: for example, assaying for antigen by its power to inhibit the combination between standard antibody and labeled antigen (Fig. 2.4b).

2.2.2 Protection

Given an antigen which has some measurable effect when injected into an experimental animal, for example, an infectious organism or toxin which can kill a mouse or a rabbit, one can assay for the corresponding antibody by the method described in Section 2.1. Specific antibody, when mixed with the antigenic agent, may neutralize it, i.e., destroy its infective power (how it does so is discussed further in Chapter 13). The titers of different antisera can be compared. Obviously this test, like most others, may be reversed and used as an assay for antigen by measuring the extent of neutralization of a standard antiserum. For example, it can be used to diagnose a particular virus in a crude isolate from an infected animal.

2.2.3 Precipitation

Under certain conditions a mixture of soluble antigen and antibody may form a precipitate. The initial combination between the two kinds of molecule occurs very rapidly; this may be followed over hours or days by the gradual appearance of a hazy precipitate in the medium caused by the formation of giant aggregates (antigen–antibody complexes) which literally fall out of solution.

Figure 2.5 explains what is happening. Most antibodies are divalent, that is, they have two identical sites at which they can combine with antigen. Antigens vary from small "monovalent" molecules to whole cells with thousands of points at which antibody may attach. Figure 2.5 shows an antigen capable of binding to four antibody combining sites. If antibody concentration is kept constantly high while antigen is increased, one will first encounter a zone of "antibody excess" where all antigen molecules are surrounded by antibody, preventing cross-linking (Ag_1Ab_x, and here $x = 4$). As more antigen is added, a zone of optimal proportions or equivalence is reached where three-dimensional aggregates or lattices of various sizes may form (Ag_yAb_y). In tubes where the antigen concentration is very high, such aggregates do not appear, because each antibody combining site is occupied by a separate antigen molecule (Ag_2Ab_1). Ultracentrifugation studies have confirmed the existence of these different kinds of complex. In recent years, it has also been possible to see them with the electron microscope.

The ability of antigen and antibody to combine in variable proportions was very puzzling to immunochemists in the early part of the century since there was no known precedent for such fickle molecular behavior. However, careful

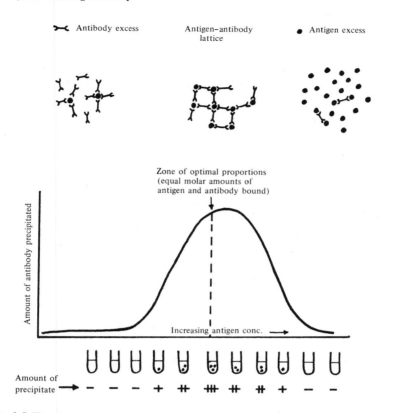

Fig. 2.5 The precipitation reaction between antigen and antibody. Precipitation occurs in a zone where antigen and antibody are present in approximately equivalent amounts. On either side of this region the complexes remain small and soluble. The perpendicular line represents the equivalence point (see Section 2.2.3).

studies of precipitation reactions by Heidelberger and his associates in the 1930's (see Table 1.1) led to the lattice hypothesis of Marrack, and to diagrams such as Fig. 2.5 which made it plain how large molecules could interact in different proportions through definite and specific bonds. The simple scheme just described is complicated, in practice, by other factors, particularly by heterogeneity of antibody (Section 2.3.4); however, it is sufficient to convey the basic principles.

2.2.4 Precipitation in Gels

This technique is widely used because it is a simple way of extracting a great deal of information about an antigen–antibody system. In the double-diffusion

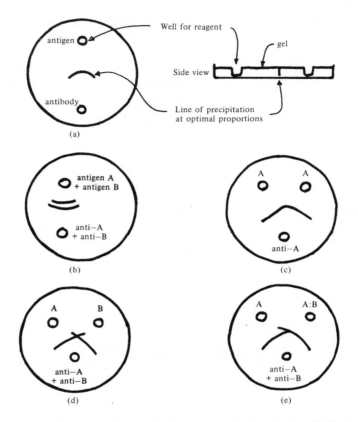

Fig. 2.6 Double-diffusion test for detecting immune precipitation in gels. (a) Single antigen–antibody band; (b) two separate reactions; (c) line of identity between two antigens reacting with the same antiserum; (d) nonidentity; (e) partial identity (see Section 2.2.4).

version devised by Ouchterlony, antigen and antibody diffuse from wells through a gel matrix (Fig. 2.6). Concentration gradients are set up, the amounts of each reagent diminishing with distance from the well. Where they meet at optimal proportions a precipitation band forms. The band is closer to that well whose reagent is least concentrated, and it is curved toward the higher molecular weight compound of the two (because this diffuses more slowly). Multiple bands may form between wells containing mixtures of different antigens and antibodies. A simple test for antigen identity is to set up two wells containing the antigens against a single serum well: a continuous line will form as in Fig. 2.6 part (c). If the antigens are different, the lines cross since each reaction takes place independently of the others. (Note that a line of "identity" means only that the same antibody molecules react with similar determinants on both antigens; this does not mean necessarily that these antigens are chemically identical.) Part (e) of the Fig. 2.6 shows an interesting pattern: the antibody well contains different antibodies to antigens A and B. One antigen well contains A alone, the other has A and B *coupled together* chemically. Here the A/anti-A reaction gives a smooth curve as in (c), while the B/anti-B precipitation takes place along a line which is not influenced by anything diffusing from well A. A "spur" or pattern indicating partial identity, results.

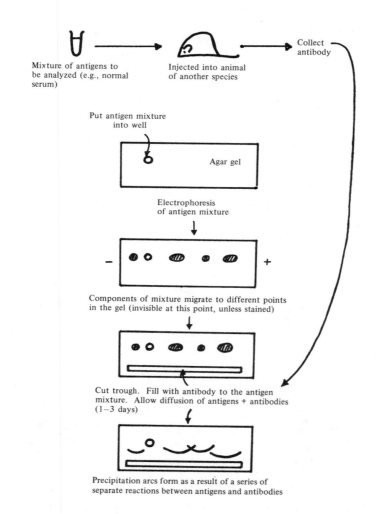

Mixture of antigens to be analyzed (e.g., normal serum)

Injected into animal of another species

Collect antibody

Put antigen mixture into well

Agar gel

Electrophoresis of antigen mixture

Components of mixture migrate to different points in the gel (invisible at this point, unless stained)

Cut trough. Fill with antibody to the antigen mixture. Allow diffusion of antigens + antibodies (1—3 days)

Precipitation arcs form as a result of a series of separate reactions between antigens and antibodies

Fig. 2.7 Immunoelectrophoresis. Components of a mixture of antigens are first separated by migration in an electric field, and are then allowed to react with antibodies against the mixture.

Variants of this technique have been developed. A particularly useful one, called immunoelectrophoresis (Fig. 2.7), involves first electrophoresing a mixture of antigens to separate them in a gel, then allowing them to react with antibody to the mixture which diffuses from a broad trough. By this technique, more than forty antigenically different components can be distinguished in normal serum.

2.2.5 Agglutination

Agglutination differs from precipitation in that antibodies are allowed to clump together large and already insoluble particles into still larger aggregates. Red blood cells are the most common type of antigenic particle used, in which case we speak of "hemagglutination." These can be clumped within minutes by specific antibody, and will settle to the bottom of the tube to form characteristic dispersed patterns visible to the naked eye. The red cells may also act as a useful indicator of antibody to other antigens which are first coupled to their surface (Fig. 2.8). Variations of the technique are again obvious: for example, inhibition of agglutination by free antigen. An interesting variation is the Coombs or antiglobulin test, where the antigen coating the cells is itself an antibody which is unable to agglutinate them by itself. These globulin-coated free red cells may be finally agglutinated by adding anti-globulin antibody, that is, anti-antibody. This last test is used clinically to detect antibody on the erythrocytes of patients with autoimmune hemolytic anemia (Section 12.3).

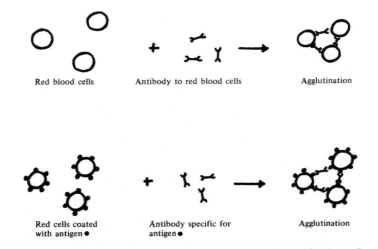

| Red blood cells | Antibody to red blood cells | Agglutination |

| Red cells coated with antigen ● | Antibody specific for antigen ● | Agglutination |

Fig. 2.8 Hemagglutination. Red cells are clumped by specific antibody. If cells are first coated with another antigen they become susceptible to agglutination by the specific antibody to this new antigen.

2.2.6 Hemolysis and Complement

The serum of normal animals of many species contains a group of at least eleven protein factors making up what is called the *complement* system. This series of substances is "activated" by complexes of antigen with certain kinds of antibody. Combination of antigen and antibody leads to a structural change in the antibody molecule, a change which is recognized by one of the components of complement. A cascade reaction begins, activation of one member of the chain leading to activation of many more of the next in line (discussed further in Section 13.1.1.4). The end result of the cascade, when it takes place on a cell surface, is that the phospholipase activity of one of the final activated components of complement punches a microscopic hole in the plasma membrane. A red blood cell, replete with hemoglobin, can be almost instantaneously converted into a "ghost" as its contents escape. This hemolysis can be observed under the microscope. If complement is added to a test system in which antibody has bound to a red blood cell, lysis or breakdown of the cells may be observed. Certain bacteria may also be destroyed in this way.

An extension of this idea is exploited in the "complement fixation" test, beloved of serologists. An antigen is mixed with serum believed to contain the corresponding antibody. If it does, the complex formed may "fix" or consume complement which is added (usually in the form of a standard dose of fresh or specially preserved guinea pig serum; any complement in the serum under test is first destroyed by heating at 56°C). The extent to which complement has been consumed can now be assessed by adding red cells coated with antibody. These fail to lyse if complement has already been "fixed," but will lyse if there was no antibody in the original serum. Complement technology enjoys a chapter to itself in Weir's book (Ref. 2.7).

2.3 SPECIFICITY AND DIVERSITY OF ANTIBODY

2.3.1 The Antibody-Combining Site

Antibody molecules have two or more combining sites (Chapter 3), regions of the molecule which bind to parts of the corresponding antigen molecules. These sites have been shown by X-ray crystallography to be cavities or clefts, which vary from one antibody to another in their three-dimensional shape and in the nature of the eight to twelve amino acids which line them. A region of antigen with a shape complementary to an antibody combining site will fit into it, the strength of the attraction depending on the distribution of charged and hydrophobic groups on the two reactants. The participants are held together not by covalent bonds, but by intermolecular forces which are similar to those involved in other protein interactions such as enzyme–substrate binding (mainly electrostatic interactions, e.g., hydrogen bonds and van der Waal's forces). The strength of the bond depends on how closely the two surfaces are apposed.

An antigenic *determinant* is that small part of an antigen which combines with a particular antibody combining site. Different antibody molecules will "see" different parts of an antigen as their corresponding antigenic determinant or region of best fit. Figure 2.9 shows an example: antibody C combines with the region of the surface of the protein antigen between A and B, while antibody D fits better between X and Y. The antigenic determinant is slighly different for each, although in both cases it contains the exposed phenol group. Obviously a determinant is not an entity which can be specified completely in isolation: like an antigen it needs to be defined in relation to the antibodies to which it binds.

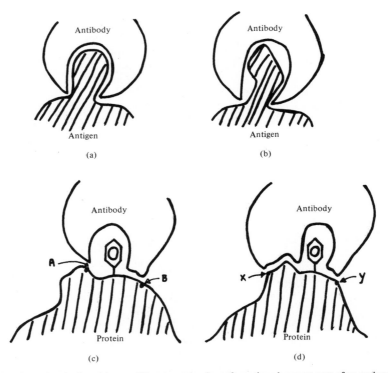

Fig. 2.9 Antigenic determinants. Diagrammatic view of reactions between part of an antigen (the "antigenic determinant") and antibody. (a) Shows a close fit, resulting in high affinity of binding; (b) a poorer fit, with lower binding affinity; (c) and (d) show the same phenolic group coupled in the same way to a protein. The antibody in (c) is reacting with that part of the protein + phenol surface which extends from A to B: a different antibody in (d) "sees" a slightly different section of the surface, X to Y (Section 2.3.1).

The size of the combining cavity has been measured by inhibition of antigen–antibody binding with antigen fragments of various sizes. For example, combination of dextran with anti-dextran antibody can be inhibited by glucose oligomers; those with six units or more are the most efficient, while shorter chains do not inhibit completely. Similar experiments with peptides show that the antibody combining site will accommodate about five amino acids. Not all groups of, say, five amino acids in a protein will be equally accessible to antibody, however; those groups most accessible tend to be "immunodominant," that is, to provoke a relatively large proportion of the antibody response.

2.3.2 Haptens

These are small molecular weight compounds which cannot induce an antibody response by themselves but can combine with antibody once it is formed. Typical examples, often used in current immunological research, are DNP (dinitrophenol) and NIP (nitroiodophenol).

These compounds will not induce antibody if injected alone. If either is coupled covalently to a foreign protein "carrier" and the conjugate injected into an animal, antibodies will be produced, some of which will combine with the hapten. This may be simply shown with an inhibition test as seen in Fig. 2.4 and described in Section 2.2.1. DNP protein is injected into an animal, where it induces antibody formation. A standard reaction is now set up between this antibody and labeled DNP protein. Excess unlabeled DNP will inhibit some of this binding, indicating the presence of antibody able to bind specifically to the DNP group. Not all of the binding will be inhibited and, in fact, most may not be, since many of the antibody molecules will combine with parts of the protein other than the hapten. The dinitrophenol could be said here to be acting as an extra antigenic determinant on the protein. The word "determinant" must be used with care: it seems to imply that the detailed fine structure ("determinant composition") is what "determines" which antibodies are formed. We will see as we learn more about the immune system that this is only one of the many factors influencing the course of an immune response (see Chapter 11).

2.3.3 Affinity and Avidity

The *affinity* of an antigen–antibody combination is an exact chemical parameter which refers to the strength of the binding between one antibody combining site and a monovalent (low molecular weight) antigen. It may be measured by various standard chemical techniques, for example, equilibrium dialysis. Each complex has, like any other noncovalently bonded system, a finite rate of dissociation into its components:

$$Ag + Ab \rightleftharpoons AgAb$$

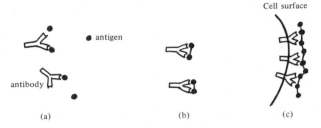

Fig. 2.10 Affinity and avidity. In (a) we have bonds between monovalent antigen and one of the combining sites of an antibody molecule. The *affinity* of this union can be measured. In (b) is shown the simultaneous combination of both valencies of an antibody molecule with two similar antigenic determinants linked together. Here we would speak of the *avidity* of antigen-antibody combination. It would be much stronger than the bonds in (a) (and could be as much as 10^4-fold stronger); when one of the two arms of antibody "lets go" the other is likely to "hold on," so overall dissociation rarely occurs. Section (c) shows the multivalent combination possible between a large antigen with repeating determinants and a series of "receptor" (Chapter 5) antibody molecules displayed on the surface of a cell. Even very low affinity individual bonds can lead to high avidity of overall combination in situations like this, with important consequences for immunology (Chapter 11).

The higher the affinity of an antibody, the further this equilibrium will lie to the right.

The avidity of binding is a term which is used more loosely to mean the overall strength of combination between an antigen of any size and a whole antibody molecule, or number of molecules close together on the surface of a cell (Fig. 2.10). Here two or more individual reactions may be occurring simultaneously between different parts of the antigen and different corresponding antibody combining sites. Such multipoint binding results in a very much firmer combination between antigen and antibody than is provided by binding at a single site. Affinity and related matters are thoroughly discussed by Eisen in Ref. 2.2.

2.3.4 Diversity of Antibody

The fact that an animal can make specific antibodies to an enormous range of antigens suggests that very many different antibodies are possible. Some concrete evidence for extreme antibody diversity comes from amino acid sequences of the uniform immunoglobulins made by certain tumors: different tumors almost never make the same sequence, as we will see in the next chapter. Another simple means of demonstrating the great heterogeneity of the antibody molecules is illustrated in Fig. 2.11. Isoelectric focusing is a way of characterizing a protein molecule by the position it adopts when electrophoresed along a pH gradient in a gel. It comes to rest at its isoelectric point. The method has very high resolution and can distinguish proteins whose isoelectric points differ by as little as 0.02 pH units. From a serum treated in this way, one can identify antibodies of a particu-

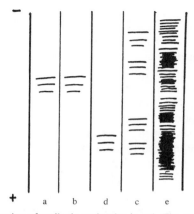

Fig. 2.11 Isoelectric focusing of antibody molecules in gel. The proteins in the serum are first brought to their isoelectric point in a pH gradient by electrophoresis. Specific antibodies are then revealed by adding low MW labeled antigen, usually radioisotope labeled material. This enters the gel and combines with the antibody bands. Uncombined antigen is now washed away, and bound antigen can be revealed by autoradiography (Section 4.9), that is, by allowing the emissions from the radioisotope to strike a sensitive overlaying emulsion. (a),(b), and (c) are typical patterns formed by single molecular species of antibody. (The multiple bands are thought to be caused by deamidation of some molecules in the serum.) These patterns are reproducible: (a) and (b) represent different samples of the same antibody; (c) is a different antibody; (d) is a pattern showing a few different products while (e) is the kind of diverse pattern often seen when whole serum is taken from an animal.

lar specificity by reacting the gel with labeled antigen, as explained in Fig. 2.11. This method has shown that there exist many hundreds of different antibodies to even a simple hapten.

It is important to realize that an antigen does not induce only accurately complementary antibodies, like wax impressions of a key (as was previously thought); it stimulates instead a spread of different antibodies with varying degrees of "goodness-of-fit." Even a chemically simple and pure antigen will usually provoke a heterogeneous response, and one which differs in different individuals. The reasons for this *degeneracy* of immune responses are complex, and are discussed further in Chapter 11. For the present we can understand what is probably the most important factor by referring again to Fig. 2.10. Antibody is produced by specialized cells (Section 4.5) which bear, on their surface, copies of their eventual product. Induction of an antigen-binding cell to produce antibody occurs under certain conditions when the cell-antigen bond is sufficiently strong (Chapter 5). Weak individual bonds, multiplied together, provide a firm overall attachment. An antigen can stimulate cells whose surface antibody "receptors" have very little individual affinity for that antigen. Under the right conditions, antigen of one kind may stimulate many cells.

2.3.5 Fine Specificity and Cross-Reactivity of Antibody

Having deliberately stressed the heterogeneity and degeneracy of antibody responses (points not usually emphasized) we must now return to a much better known and very useful property of antibody molecules, their specificity. "Specificity" means the ability of an antibody or antiserum to react with one antigen and not with another. The work of Landsteiner in the 1930's brought some precision to the concept of antibody specificity by showing just what very small changes antibody can detect in an antigen molecule. A favorite example is shown in Fig. 2.12. Antibody induced by *m*-aminobenzoate hapten coupled to protein reacted much less strongly to ortho and para isomers, or to molecules with other side groups in the meta position, and not at all to the other variants shown. It seems that the shape of the determinant cannot be greatly changed without reducing the strength of binding to a particular antibody.

This example also shows that antibody initially induced by one antigenic determinant will, however, cross-react with certain others which are similar. There are two reasons for this: (1) Antibodies which combine with X may also be able to accommodate Y, much as shown in Fig. 2.9. This is clearly the case when entirely homogeneous antibodies (for example, those obtained from myelomas;

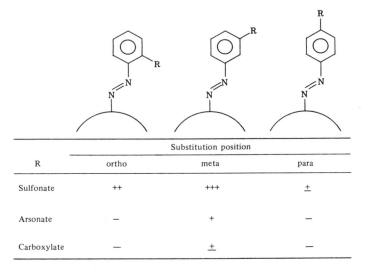

R	Substitution position		
	ortho	meta	para
Sulfonate	++	+++	±
Arsonate	−	+	−
Carboxylate	−	±	−

Fig. 2.12 Specificity and cross-reactivity of antibody. Antibodies were raised to the *m*-aminobenzene sulfonate hapten coupled to a protein. The above 9 different haptens were tested for their ability to inhibit a standard precipitation reaction between the immunizing hapten and its antiserum. The effect of substitution of different side groups in different positions on the hapten is scored according to its inhibitory effect on the precipitation: + + + strong; − none.

Section 3.1) combine with more than one antigen. (2) An anti-X antiserum will also almost always contain a heterogeneous mixture of antibodies, as discussed in the last section, some with high affinity for X, and some with low. A proportion of these may combine as well or even better with another antigen, Y, than with the immunizing antigen X (such "heteroclitic" antibodies have been observed experimentally).

We should summarize the last two sections and attempt to reconcile the two rather opposite properties of antibody, its specificity and its degeneracy. Individual antibody molecules from an animal immunized with X usually bind more strongly to X than to chemically related antigens, and the strength of binding decreases to become undetectable by conventional tests against most second randomly selected antigens. When we consider whole antiserum from an animal immunized with X, the same rule is broadly true, but we should bear in mind that a serum is the sum of many components, and be prepared to find that different sera cross-react to varying extents with related antigens. The pattern seen in Fig. 2.12 is not reproduced exactly by all immune sera.

Having digested this, we can consider a final complication. Most antigens are complex. Antigen ABCD, by provoking antibodies to all parts of itself, will naturally yield an antiserum which cross-reacts with antigen ABEF. Cross-reactions (binding of the same antibody) by what appear to be very different proteins may occur because they share small regions with very similar or identical shapes. Some of the subtleties of immune specificity and degeneracy are pursued in Ref. 2.1.

2.4 PROTECTIVE IMMUNITY

It has been known for thousands of years in many human societies that recovery from epidemic diseases may confer immunity. Edward Jenner took knowledge a step further in 1796 when he showed that the deliberate infection of people with cowpox, a relatively mild infection, would protect these individuals from subsequent exposure to the related, but much more virulent, organism of smallpox. He is said to have realized that milkmaids as a group were usually spared the ravages of smallpox because of their contact with the milder disease,

> Where are you going to my *pretty* maid?
> I'm going a milking, Sir, she said

and a face unmarked by pocks was more likely to be a pretty one. The word *vaccination* comes from *vacca* (*Latin,* a cow). Cowpox virus is now called vaccinia. Louis Pasteur put vaccination into a rational and general framework when he demonstrated that chicken cholera, anthrax, and rabies organisms could be deliberately *attenuated* or weakened in virulence by growing them in certain ways, before using them as a vaccine. Today, of course, vaccination, or treatment with relatively harmless organisms or products as a method for inducing future immunity against disease, is a routine and important procedure in many countries (see Chapter 12).

Active immunization is the process of acquiring resistance to infectious disease by natural exposure or vaccination. (As we have seen, the word is extended to also cover development of reactivity to noninfectious antigens whether encountered naturally or artificially administered.) First contact with antigen induces a *primary immune response* during which free antibody is circulating in the body fluids and can neutralize invading organisms or their product. It also induces a state of *memory* which we have mentioned already and will discuss further in Chapter 6. The individual, therefore, is "primed" and able to give a more rapid *secondary response* to a subsequent exposure to the same antigen. This state may last long after the antibody from the primary response has declined. So we have two distinct phases in active immunity, the production of the protective mechanisms (e.g., antibody) for a relatively short period, followed by the long-lasting latent state of memory. "Immunization" usually refers to the establishing in an animal of this second, memory state.

If antibodies protect, we would expect to be able to transfer a state of immunity *passively* from an animal with a high titer in its serum to a normal recipient animal (Fig. 2.1). This was first demonstrated by von Behring in 1891 when he saved the life of a child dying of diphtheria by injecting her with serum from a previously immunized sheep. Another familiar example is the routine injection of antibodies to tetanus toxin into people with deep wounds. Such passive immunity is immediate—the antibodies can get to work immediately in their new host. It is also transient (lasting for several weeks only), because the transferred antibody gradually decays. The animal's own immune system is not actively involved, so no state of memory results.

A third and naturally important example of passive immunity is the transmission of antibody in mammals from mother to offspring. The fetus is normally not exposed to foreign antigens during gestation, and it makes very little antibody globulin, relying on antibody from the mother for early protection after birth. This maternal antibody is transmitted across the placenta in some species, and to a variable extent in the milk of all species examined. Where the placenta is multilayered, as, for example, in ruminants, no antibody can pass through it, but for the first few days of life the gut of the young animal has the power to absorb directly the globulins present in large amounts in the "colostrum," or first milk made by the mother during lactation. In humans, most antibody crosses via the placenta: the small globulin molecules (IgG and not IgM or IgA; see Section 3.2) are selectively transmitted. In mice, both routes are important.

We can see now that a state of immunity implies a comparison with a less responsive state. Immunity, in this biological sense, is an adaptation of a particular kind to the environment. Immunology began as a study of the development of acquired immunity to infectious organisms. Its scope has now broadened enormously, to include responses to noninfectious and synthetic antigens, graft rejection (Chapter 10), autoimmune disease (Chapter 12), hypersensitivity states (Chapters 9 and 12), and some reactions to neoplasms (Chapter 14).

2.5 SUMMARY

Antigens are substances, usually foreign to an animal, which stimulate an *immune response*. The best studied kind of response involves production of *antibodies*, serum gamma-globulins which combine specifically with the immunizing antigen. During an immune response *titers* (levels) of specific antibody may rise many thousandfold, as can be demonstrated by a variety of serological tests.

Antibodies have specific *combining sites* (usually two per molecule). These are clefts formed by the folding of the molecule in defined regions. These sites combine noncovalently with small regions of the antigen (*determinants*: about five amino acids in size) which have complementary shape and can "fit into" the cleft. Serum from an immunized animal usually contains a great array of different antibody molecules with different *affinities* (binding power) for various regions on the antigen. Such sera can be very *specific*, i.e., react more strongly with the immunizing antigen than with chemically related but different compounds.

FURTHER READING

2.1   Cunningham, A. J. (1974). "Predicting What Antibodies an Antigen will Induce: The Inadequacy of the Determinant Theory," *Curr. Top. Microbiol. Immunol.* **67**, 97. Further discussion of immune degeneracy.

2.2   Davis, B. D., Dulbecco, R., Eisen, H. N., Ginsberg, H. S., and Wood, W. B. (1973), "Microbiology." Harper International Edition (2nd ed.). Includes an immunology section which is particularly strong on immunochemical aspects.

2.3   Gell. P. H., Coombs, R. R. A., and Lachmann, P. J. (1975). "Clinical Aspects of Immunology." Blackwell Scientific Publ., Oxford.

2.4   Hudson, L. and Hay, F. C. (1975). "Practical Immunology." Blackwell Scientific Publ., Oxford.

2.5   Kabat, E. A. (1968). "Structural Concepts in Immunology and Immunochemistry." Holt, Rinehart and Winston, Inc., New York. An introduction to immunochemistry.

2.6   Landsteiner K. (1945). "The Specificity of Serological Reactions," 2nd ed. Harvard Univ. Press, Cambridge, Massachusetts. A classical work.

2.7   Weir, D. M. (1974). "Handbook of Experimental Immunology," 2nd ed. Blackwell Scientific Publ., Oxford. Descriptions of common immunological techniques.

QUESTIONS

2.1   Serum was collected from a rabbit injected with 10^9 killed *Salmonella abortus-equi* organisms. The serum had an agglutination titer of 1/10,000: what does this statement mean? The same serum agglutinated other bacteria of types A, B, and C to titers of 1/7500, 1/100, and 1/2, respectively. What can you deduce about the possible relationships of A, B, and C to the original immunizing strain of bacteria?

2.2   Antisera against a foreign protein was made in two different rabbits. An antigen-binding assay (Section 2.2.1) was set up using radioactively labeled antigen which was allowed to react with antibody, the complexes then being precipitated with ammonium sulfate. To a standard amount of each serum, an exactly equivalent amount of labeled antigen was added, i.e., all of the label and all of the specific antibody were precipitated. It was found, however, that some label remained in the supernatant if excess unlabeled antigen was added to the initial antigen-antibody mixture and left in the tube for several hours before salt precipitation. Why? Ten times more unlabeled antigen had to be added to one tube than to the other to recover the same amount of supernatant radioactivity: what difference does this indicate between the two antisera?

2.3   If, to a constant amount of specific antiserum (antitoxin), an exactly equivalent amount of diphtheria toxin is added, the mixture becomes nontoxic. If, however, the same amount of toxin is added in two fractions with an interval of more than 15 minutes between additions, the mixture remains toxic; this is called the Danysz phenomenon. Can you explain it? (Hint: see Fig. 2.5.)

2.4   What conclusions might you draw from the finding that a rabbit- anti-human globulin antibody agglutinated the red blood cells of some, but not all humans?

Molecular Biology of Antibody Formation

The diversity of antibody function turns out to be based on a corresponding degree of diversity in the primary amino acid sequences of the antibody molecules themselves. This is perhaps what one would have expected given modern knowledge of protein synthesis and structure. However, as we shall see in Chapter 7, it was believed for many years that antibody variability might come from folding the same basic molecule in many ways around different antigen templates. Immunoglobulin structural studies have been helpful in dispelling this myth. They have also provided molecular explanations for many of the functions of antibodies. But perhaps their main relevance for immunological theory has been the fierce controversy which knowledge of antibody sequences has provoked about the underlying genetic basis of antibody variability. This debate continues.

What follows is a summary of modern views on immunoglobulin (Ig) structure. There is no escaping the fact that this is a complex area, and one which may prove confusing to some newcomers. A detailed knowledge of Ig genetics and structure is perhaps not essential for understanding the rest of immunology, but it is important to emerge from the present chapter with a firm grasp of the following five points:

(a) Most antibodies have four polypeptide chains, two identical "light" and two identical "heavy."

(b) Each chain has a constant region, and also a variable region whose amino acid sequence differs greatly from one antibody molecule to another.

(c) Constant and variable regions are coded for by separate genes, but the whole polypeptide chain containing both regions is translated from a single RNA message.

(d) Every animal has only a small number of genes for constant regions of its immunoglobulins, and a very large number for the variable regions.

(e) It is currently debatable whether the variable-region genes all exist in germline (gamete) DNA and in every cell of the body, or whether these genes are created by somatic events from a small initial number as each individual develops (see Section 3.6).

3.1 GROSS STRUCTURE OF IgG. MYELOMAS

The immunoglobulins (Ig) are a heterogeneous group of proteins which migrate electrophoretically in the globulin region of serum (Fig. 2.2). They include known antibodies and molecules with similar structure but of unknown activity. By immunoelectrophoresis (Fig. 2.7), it is easy to show a number of precipitation arcs among these proteins; evidently they vary both in migratory properties and in antigenicity. (Like any other large molecules, immunoglobulins may themselves act as antigens to another species. "Anti-antibodies" can be used to distinguish different antigenic and hence molecular types of Ig.) The major immunoglobulin component of serum (about 75%) may be separated from albumin by precipitation in high salt concentrations and purified further by chromatography on ion-exchange columns. It is called immunoglobulin G or IgG, and has a molecular weight of about 150,000. This material is still far from homogeneous by physicochemical criteria; for example, it will not crystallize.

Chemical studies by Edelman and by Porter suggested the structure of IgG which is shown in Fig. 3.1. Each molecule has two heavy or H chains (MW ~50,000) and two light or L chains (25,000). They are held together by disulfide bridges and by noncovalent forces. Reduction with mercaptoethanol can be used to separate L and H chains. The proteolytic enzyme papain splits the molecule into an Fc (crystallizable) fragment and two Fab fragments. These latter fragments retain antigen binding power, but will not precipitate antigen. Thus, an Fab piece, which is made up of one L chain and about one-half of an H chain, includes only one of the two antibody combining sites of the originally bivalent molecule. Another proteolytic enzyme, pepsin, cleaves the molecule in a slightly different position as shown in the figure, yielding a divalent $F(ab')_2$ unit which can still precipitate antigen. Isolated L and H chains have relatively little ability to bind antigen: it appears that the combining site uses a part of both H and L chains. Electron microscopic examination of purified IgG molecules confirm that they have a Y shape, some flexibility in the angle of the Y being imparted by a number of proline residues at the papain/pepsin-sensitive *hinge* region.

Our knowledge of the structure of antibodies has increased dramatically with the discovery of tumors (called *myelomas*) of antibody forming cells. As with other neoplasms it seems that a myeloma develops when a single (mutant?) cell escapes from normal physiological controls and proliferates wildly, often causing death of the host. Such tumors are responsible for a group of diseases in man, and

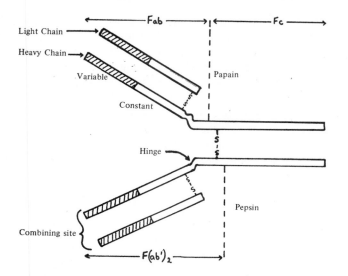

Fig. 3.1 The basic four-chain structure of IgG (see also Fig. 3.5). (There are species and subclass differences in the number and position of disulfide bridges.) Papain digestion produces two identical Fab subunits, while pepsin leaves these joined as a divalent F(ab')$_2$ which has agglutinating power. The two L chains are identical in any one molecule, as are the two H. The molecule is shown diagrammatically as four rigid chains, but in reality these are extensively folded. Flexibility at the hinge region probably allows the two combining sites to interact with two identical antigenic determinants spaced at varying distances from one another.

may also be induced in some strains of mice by injecting certain mineral oils. Their importance to basic immunology is that they are a source of Ig from a single *clone* of cells, i.e., a large number of cells all of which are descendants of one initial (antibody producing) ancestor. For this reason (see also Chapter 4), the Ig is usually homogeneous. It has two identical H and two identical L chains, and may often be crystallized, in marked contrast to normal serum IgG which is always the heterogeneous product of many clones. Myeloma proteins may be collected in large amounts from serum. In addition, some human patients secrete homogeneous L chains (called Bence-Jones proteins after their discoverer) into their urine. *In vitro* cell lines are now available which also produce a single molecular species of Ig.

Myeloma protein, being relatively pure, may be sequenced, and we will discuss the amino acid composition of Ig molecules shortly. For the moment, we should note that from Bence-Jones and myeloma proteins it has been found that there are two types of light chains, called κ (kappa) and λ (lambda). The actual experimental operations behind this statement are of the following kind. If, for example, a rabbit is immunized with Bence-Jones protein from a single human patient, an antiserum may be raised which reacts with that L chain, and with L chains from many other, but not all, similar patients. All L chains reacting with the antiserum might be said to be of the κ antigenic type. Similarly, all other non-κ L chains are found to fall into a second antigenic group, λ type. Normal serum IgG contains a mixture of molecules, some reacting with anti-κ, and the rest with anti-λ. This classification, initially based on antigenic differences between κ and λ chains, has since been shown to depend on systematic differences in amino acid sequence between the two kinds of L chain. The proportion of total Ig molecules with either type varies from one species to another: humans have 2κ:1λ, mice have nearly all κ, and horses nearly all λ. In any one Ig molecule, both L chains are the same.

3.2 OTHER Ig CLASSES

Besides IgG there are four other *classes* of immunoglobulin recognized in man: IgM, IgA, IgD, and IgE. (Similar class heterogeneity occurs in mice, and other species. We will discuss man here.) These other classes all use exactly the same L chains, κ and λ, but each has a characteristic heavy chain type. For the five classes, G, M, A, D, and E, these heavy or H chains are called γ, μ, α, δ, and ϵ. Myelomas exist for all these classes, and may be used to classify immunoglobulins in exactly the same way as L chains were divided into their two categories. For example, an antiserum is made against IgG from a myeloma. This contains anti-L and anti-H chain antibodies. The anti-L are absorbed, perhaps by passing the serum through a column containing purified L chains coupled to an insoluble support. The residual anti-H chain antibody now reacts with γ chains but fails to react with the product of some other myelomas, which are provisionally classified as having a different H chain. Reciprocal sera are prepared and tested. Eventually the classification is strengthened by examining other properties of the two H chains, such as molecular weight and amino acid sequence.

Some liberties have been taken with history to make it clear in principle how different Ig classes may be distinguished. In fact, IgM, the second most prevalent class, was separated very early by ultracentrifugation from IgG by Heidelberger, who found antibody activity in both rapidly and slowly sedimenting molecular classes from serum. IgM has a molecular weight of about 900,000, and consists of five units, each the approximate size of IgG, joined together as shown in Fig. 3.2. It is important to note that IgM is *not* simply five IgG molecules joined together: the two classes, while using the same L chains, have different H chains. All Ig molecules contain some carbohydrate: IgM molecules have 12% as opposed to only 3% for IgG. An IgM molecule has a valency of ten when reacting with small haptens, but quantitative antigen binding measurements with larger antigens often detect only five, probably for reasons of steric restriction, i.e., all of the sites can not attach to the same antigenic structure at the same time.

IgA is the other class found in moderate amounts. It exists usually as dimers and as higher polymers bound together by a 16,000 MW polypeptide called the J (joining) chain (Fig. 3.2). Some properties of the different Ig classes are shown in Table 3.1.

Why this multiplicity of classes? We can think of an antibody molecule as having two distinct parts, its combining sites, and the attached Fc portion(s). The Fc structure influences the biological activity of the molecule: different classes have different distributions in the body and different properties. The combining sites obviously determine what antigens are bound, and the rest of the molecule controls what happens to the antigen–antibody complex. In addition, the act of combination may induce changes in the Fc portion which can give rise to altered activities. For example, free antibody molecules do not bind complement, while antibodies of M and G classes, when complexed with antigen, do bind complement via their Fc regions.

IgM is the first antibody to be made in most immune responses. With its large molecular weight, it is confined mainly to the bloodstream where its high valency makes it a good agglutinator of foreign particles. Deficiency of IgM is often associated with susceptibility to septicemia. IgG, being smaller, diffuses more readily into extravascular spaces. It is also selectively transported across the placenta of primates, and can confer passive immunity (Section 2.4) on the infant after birth. As the predominant species of Ig, it is the class most responsible for

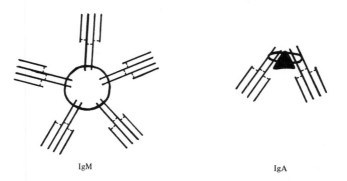

IgM   IgA

Fig. 3.2 Gross structure of IgM and IgA molecules. Dotted lines represent disulfide linkages. IgA exists both as monomers and polymers (a dimer is shown). The monomeric units of IgM and of IgA are linked into stable polymeric forms by a small (MW approximately 16,000) cysteine-rich polypeptide, produced by the antibody-forming cell, and called the J (joining) chain. It is shown here diagrammatically as a circle or ellipse. There is one J chain per polymer. IgA in external secretions (gut, saliva, milk) carries an additional polypeptide chain, the secretory piece (MW approx. 60,000) shown here as a triangular structure. It is synthesized by epithelial cells and attached to the IgA as the latter is secreted. Its function may be to protect the molecule from degradation.

neutralizing bacterial toxins and binding to invading microorganisms. Both IgG and IgM act as opsonins, that is, when bound to microorganisms they enhance the palatability of the latter to macrophages and other phagocytic scavenger cells (see Sections 4.2.4 and 13.1.1.3), which then digest the invaders. Both classes also fix complement, and can thus directly lyse bacteria (Section 2.2.6).

IgA appears selectively in seromucous secretions such as saliva, tears, nasal fluids, and secretions of the lung and gastrointestinal tract. It seems to have the job of protecting these surfaces of the body against attack by microorganisms. It is synthesized locally, and has a secretory or transport piece (Fig. 3.2) added during its passage into mucous secretions from the lamina propria. This addition apparently makes the molecule less susceptible to digestion by proteolytic enzymes.

The function of IgD (discovered through recognition of a myeloma protein with a new H chain) is still uncertain. There are recent indications that it has a specialized role as a cell receptor (Section 5.2.3). IgE antibodies bind, via their Fc part, to mast cells in skin and in other tissues. When antigen then combines with the free Fab parts of these cell-bound molecules, the mast cells degranulate, releasing pharmacologically active factors such as histamine. These factors are responsible for symptoms of such allergic conditions (Chapter 12) as hay fever and extrinsic asthma when the patient comes in contact with the antigen to which he is sensitive (i.e., against which he has IgE antibody). Whether IgE has a beneficial role is uncertain; its level increases in some metazoan parasitic infections, and it may help in rejecting such parasites.

TABLE 3.1
Properties of Human Ig Classes[a]

	IgG	IgM	IgA	IgD	IgE
H chain	γ	μ	α	δ	ϵ
Molecular formula[b]	$\gamma_2 L_2$	$(\mu_2 L_2)_5$	$(\alpha_2 L_2)_{1-3}$	$\delta_2 L_2$	$\epsilon_2 L_2$
Molecular weight	150,000	900,000	160,000 + polymers	185,000	200,000
Sedimentation coefficient (S value)	7	19	7, 9	7	8
Valency	2	5(10)	2 or more	?	2
Concentration in normal serum (mg/ml)	8–16	0.5–2	1.4–4	0–0.4	0.0001– 0.0007
Half-life (days)[c]	23	5	6	3	3

[a] After Fudenberg *et al.* (Ref. 3.9).
[b] In all classes the L chain may be κ or λ in different molecules.
[c] The average length of time for which one half of recently synthesized Ig molecules persist in serum.

TABLE 3.2
**Diagrammatic Representation of Human
Ig Structural Genes**[a,b]

Loci for	Genes for C regions	Probable genes for V region subgroups
κ chains	κ	V_κ I
		V_κ II
		V_κ III
		V_κ IV
λ chains[c]	$\lambda_{oz}{}^+$	V_λ I
	$\lambda_{oz}{}^-$	V_λ II
		V_λ III
		V_λ IV
		V_λ V
H chains[d]	γ_1	V_H I
	γ_2	V_H II
	γ_3	V_H III
	γ_4	V_H IV
	μ	
	α_1	
	α_2	
	δ	
	ϵ	

[a] Adapted from Fudenberg *et al.* (Ref. 3.9).
[b] Each individual has all the C region genes and probably at least this number of V region genes.
[c] There is very recent evidence for the existence of more human λ chains.
[d] The complete immunoglobulin molecules containing these chains are known as IgG_1, IgG_2–IgM, etc. Mouse immunoglobulins are labeled slightly differently: the four subclasses of IgG are called IgG_1, IgG_{2a}, IgG_{2b}, and IgG_3.

Thus, at the level of gross structure, immunoglobulins fall into several classes depending on their H chains, each of which may be associated with one of two types of L chains (Table 3.2). There is one further refinement to be mentioned here. Antigenic analysis of human IgG myelomas shows that they can be further subdivided into four "subclasses." Each has a different H chain (γ_1, γ_2, γ_3, or γ_4) but the differences between them are slight (90% amino acid homology) compared with the gross differences between classes. Similarly two IgA subclasses have been reported in man. Kappa light chains all fall into one "class," while two closely similar "subclasses" of λ are known as $\lambda_{oz}{}^+$ and $\lambda_{oz}{}^-$, which differ from one another only by one amino acid.

In summary, we have identified twelve different polypeptide chains in human Ig molecules: three L chains, κ, $\lambda_{oz}{}^+$, and $\lambda_{oz}{}^-$ and nine H chains: γ_1, γ_2, γ_3, γ_4, μ, α_1, α_2, δ, and ϵ. These Ig components, classes, and subclasses, are sometimes called *isotypes:* all are present in any one individual (Table 3.2). (Recent work suggests that the number of isotypes of human λ chains may be as high as eight.)

3.3 ALLOTYPES

The fact that there are at least twelve types of Ig polypeptide chains implies that there must be a corresponding number of different genes in each individual. How are these genes arranged in the cell DNA? For example, are they all present on the same chromosome and in one linked group?

We can move from proteins to genes by considering genetic variants or markers which exist on the Ig chains. If an individual homozygous for the κ chain gene suffers a (harmless) mutation at this locus in a germinal cell, he may pass on to his different offspring one of two types of genes, differing by one base pair, which code for two recognizably different κ chains. Let us call these A and B. They may be distinguished antigenically, or by sequencing amino acids, or in some other way. These new kinds of κ chains may, after many generations, spread through a considerable fraction of the population. Each individual would have one or the other type of κ gene, A or B, at the κ locus in each of two chromosomes in every diploid cell. Individuals could be homozygous or heterozygous, for A or B. But any one gamete could contain only A or B, not both. They are alternative forms of the same allele, allelotypes or *allotypes.* (Similar *polymorphism* exists among the products of many loci, e.g., in blood group substances, and this kind of variation, of course, forms the pool on which natural selection acts.) *Immunogenetics* studies the inheritance and expression of such markers which are known for many Ig genes (Refs. 3.9 and 3.11).

Look now at Fig. 3.3: an animal heterozygous for the A and B allotypes of κ chains will have the A gene on one chromosome, and the B on the other. Each gamete will contain only one of these two genes. If the locus responsible for γ chains is unlinked to κ (e.g., on an entirely different chromosome) and if "W" and "X" genetic variants of γ are identifiable, then four types of gamete are possible, representing independent segregation of these two markers. All these four combinations should turn up in different offspring (together with genes from the other parent); this is found to be so. Consider now closely linked genes, like μ and γ. Genetic markers in these genes will segregate together through generations of breeding.

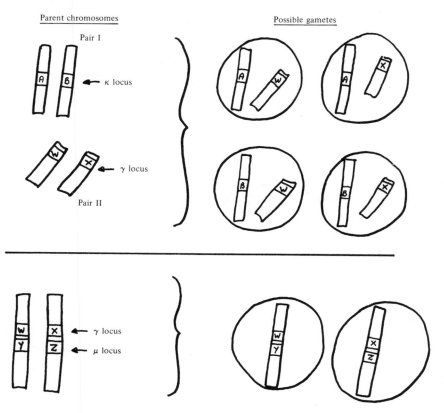

Fig. 3.3 Inheritance of genetic markers on immunoglobulins. The upper diagram shows how, when the different polypeptides are coded for at unlinked loci, they assort randomly in the gametes and are inherited independently. Where loci coding for two chains are closely linked (lower diagram), allotypes are inherited together.

This reminder of elementary genetic principles is inserted because a number of important conclusions in immunology result from its application. Immunogenetic analysis has, for example, shown that Ig chains are coded for at three separate loci, one for each light chain and one locus for the H chains: all the H chain genes form one tightly linked group. This knowledge allows us to move one step further ahead in our classification of Ig genes, as shown in Table 3.2. For the moment, only the ''C regions'' are relevant.

It must be stressed that allotypes are simply genetic markers which enable us to identify which gene comes from the father and which from the mother, and how various groups of genes are related. Unlike ''isotypes'' they are not an important additional source of heterogeneity in the individual: each person expresses only one kind of, say, κ chain, or γ^1 chain, if he is homozygous at these loci, and at most two kinds if heterozygous.

Work with allotypes has also demonstrated a unique and important property of the immune system which we will note here and discuss further in Chapter 8. Consider a man heterozygous at the γ_1 locus (Fig. 3.3). Both W and X allotypes of IgG$_1$ would be found in his serum. Individual cells, however, make only W or X, never both. This is called *allelic exclusion:* only one of two alleles is expressed at one particular locus in a diploid cell. This is true for all immunoglobulins, but not for any other known single locus in vertebrates.

3.4 AMINO ACID SEQUENCES: V REGIONS

The limited amount of heterogeneity described so far among Ig molecules obviously cannot account for the diversity of antibody specificity. The molecular basis for this diversity only became obvious when sequence studies were done on myeloma proteins (some with known antigen binding activity) and more recently on homogeneous normal antibodies induced in various ways.

Figure 3.4 compares the complete amino acid sequences of Bence–Jones proteins from two human patients. These are two different, pure, complete, λ-type L chains. The main features shown here and in large numbers of similar sequences are as follows:

1. All Ig polypeptide chains consist of two regions: an amino terminal section of the about 110 residues called the variable or V region, and a carboxy terminal portion called the constant or C region which is 110 amino acids long in L chains and three to four times this length in the larger H chains.

2. The sequence of amino acids varies extensively from one V region to the next. Among hundreds of known sequences there are very few repeats.

3. The C region is always the same within any one subclass or type (except for occasional small variations responsible for allotypes). It is this C region which defines antigenic and other properties of each class or subclass.

4. The nomenclature used is V_L = variable region of a light chain (V_κ or V_λ may be specified), C_L = constant region of L chain; V_H and C_H = analogous regions of H chains.

5. Variation within V regions does not occur at all positions. There are some constant residues, perhaps needed to assure some constancy of structure (folding). When all known V_κ regions are aligned to maximize sequence homology (small deletions in some molecules being inferred from the way the chain matches best with others on either side) it is found that any two differ by about 15–40 amino acids out of the 110. V_λ and V_H regions show similar variability.

6. All V regions associated with λ chains have some sequences of amino acids in common, and a similar rule holds for V_κ and V_H. So it appears that each

```
1                                           10                        20                                      50
PCA·Ser Val Leu Thr Gln Pro Pro Ser Val Ser Gly Thr Pro Gly Gln Arg Val Thr Ile Ser Cys Ser Gly Gly
        Ala                                                                                          Thr
            Ser                                                                                   Leu Leu Ile
                                                                                                     Val

                30                      40
Ser Ser· Asn Gly Thr Gly Asn Asn Tyr Val Tyr Trp Tyr Gln Gln Leu Pro Gly Thr Ala Pro Lys Leu Leu Ile
         Asp Val Gly Asn Asp Lys                  Ser                His                Arg             Val

                        60                      70
Tyr Arg Asp Asp Lys Arg Pro Ser Gly Val Pro Asp Arg Phe Ser Gly Ser Lys Ser Gly Thr Ser Ala Ser Leu
Phe Glu Val Ser Gln                                               Asn Asp Thr

        80                      90                     100
Ala Ile Ser Gly Leu Arg Ser Glu Asp Glu Ala Asp Tyr His Cys Ala Ala Trp Asp Tyr Arg Leu Ser Ala Val
Thr Val                              Ala    Asp           Tyr     Ser Ser Tyr Val Asp Asn Asn Phe  ?

                                    110                      120
Val Phe Gly Gly Gly Thr Gln Leu Thr Val Leu Arg Gln Pro Lys Ala Ala Pro Ser Val Thr Leu Phe Pro Pro
                                                 Lys

                        130                     140                     150
Ser Ser Glu Glu Leu Gln Ala Asn Lys Ala Thr Leu Val Cys Leu Ile Ser Asp Phe Tyr Pro Gly Ala Val Thr

                        160                     170
Val Ala Trp Lys Ala Asp Ser Ser Pro Val Lys Ala Gly Val Glu Thr Thr Thr Pro Ser Lys Gln Ser Asn Asn

                        180                     190                     200
Lys Tyr Ala Ala Ser Ser Tyr Leu Ser Leu Thr Pro Glu Gln Trp Lys Ser His Arg Ser Tyr Ser Cys Gln Val

                        210
Thr His Glu Gly Ser Thr Val Glu Lys Thr Val Ala Pro Thr Glu Cys Ser
```

Fig. 3.4 Comparison of the complete amino acid sequences of two human Bence-Jones proteins. The sequence of one protein is given in full at the top, and only the positions where the other differs in sequence are indicated. The chains are of the λ type, but similar variation between proteins is observed in κ and heavy chains. Comparison of several λ chains indicates that sequence variation in these chains is observed between positions 1 and 107 (the variable region). The remainder of the chain constitutes the constant region. PCA is pyrrolidonecarboxylic acid (a cyclized, glutamic acid derivative). (After Fudenberg et al. Ref. 3.9.)

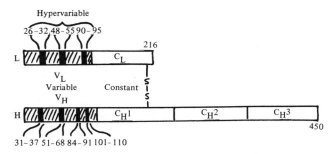

Fig. 3.5 Domains and hypervariable regions. Diagram of one L plus one H chain of a typical immunoglobulin molecule. The L chain has two domains (V_L and C_L) while the H chain has four of similar size (after Williamson, Ref. 3.17). The numbers refer to amino acids, counting from the N-terminal end of each chain.

of the three Ig loci has its own particular DNA sequences coding for V regions, not shared by the other two loci. In any H chain, whether it be μ, γ_1, γ_2, α, etc., the V region will have certain sequence characteristics which label it as belonging to the H locus, and not to either of the L loci.

The sequences in Fig. 3.4 illustrate another important feature of V regions. Amidst a highly variable terrain, "peaks" or hot spots of still greater variability (from one sequence to another) are found. There are three or four such regions per V gene, depending on the class of chain (Fig. 3.5). One might guess that the molecule is folded in such a way that these *hypervariable regions* together form the antibody combining site, combinations of regions with different sequences providing surfaces with a great variety of shapes. This has been directly demonstrated by an elegant technique called affinity labeling. Antibodies are allowed to combine with a hapten which contains a reactive group able to form a covalent link with the Ig molecule near the site of binding. The bound hapten, therefore, labels those regions of the molecule which were directly involved in the binding. When the molecule is unfolded, it can be seen that label is attached to hypervariable regions of both heavy and light chains. In recent years, X-ray crystallography applied to purified Ig has directly demonstrated the wedge-shaped cavities or clefts in which haptenic antigens become bound (Ref. 3.1).

3.5 TWO GENES, ONE POLYPEPTIDE CHAIN

The hypothesis "one gene–one enzyme" was proposed by Beadle and Tatum in 1943. One of the most remarkable things about immunoglobulins is that they seem to be an exception to this rule. *Separate* genes exist for C and V regions, and two genes are therefore involved in the synthesis of any one Ig polypeptide chain. The main argument for this is as follows: there are separate genes for the C region of each Ig class. For the H chain locus there must be at least nine different genes, closely linked, and probably in a linear array along one chromosome. Now there is evidence that single V_H regions (defined by sequence or other properties) can be found joined to more than one kind of C_H region. (In one case, for example, a single myeloma was found producing μ and γ_2 H chains each attached to the same V region). The simplest explanation is that separate pieces of DNA exist for V and C, and that one V gene may be translocated in some way to become contiguous with any one of several C genes.

Fusion of C and V regions is conceivable at three levels, DNA, messenger RNA, or protein synthesis. A joining of two preformed polypeptides seems excluded by biosynthetic studies which show that each L and each H chain is translated as a continuous chain from their amino terminal end on the polyribosomes. Ig synthesis seems in fact to follow the same rules as the production of any other differentiated cell product (Ref. 3.2). (It should be noted that H and L chains are made quite independently of one another, and the whole Ig molecule assembled in the cytoplasm. The present discussion refers only to VC joinings.) Messenger RNA molecules for whole chains, V + C, have been isolated; from these messengers Ig polypeptides can be translated in cell-free systems. It is currently believed that V and/or C genes may be translocated, perhaps by a crossing over event, or because one or the other forms an "episome" which reintegrates elsewhere in the DNA, much as a phage integrates into the genome of its bacterial host. A V gene might "travel" to, say, a site adjacent to a C_γ gene, after which a complete message VC could be transcribed. Without delving too deeply into another difficult area it can be said that allotype markers of V genes are also known (particularly in rabbits). Animals heterozygous at both H chain constant (C_H) and H chain variable (V_H) region loci show that translocation is predominantly "cis," that is, maternal C genes join to maternal and not paternal V genes at the same locus. The translocation event is probably also somehow responsible for the phenomenon of allelic exclusion mentioned in Section 8.1. It will be evident that this most interesting phenomenon is not yet fully understood. There may be some surprises in store for us.

Recapitulating, we have described three genetic loci each coding for a number of linked genes which include one or several C genes, and one or more (not yet discussed) V genes. At one locus, any V gene can translocate to combine with any of the C genes. The adjacent VC combinations are transcribed as one message.

3.6 HOW MANY V GENES?

By now we can see clearly that one of the most important immunogenetic questions is: how many V genes are there? Can something be inferred from patterns of Ig V region sequences? We shall discuss some aspects of the question here, and return to it from another point of view in Chapter 7.

Obviously many V regions mean many V genes, if one accepts that Ig proteins are transcribed and translated in the conventional way. [There is still occasionally some heretical discussion about the possibility of the following pathway:

$$\text{(Protein) antigen} \xrightarrow{\text{reverse translatase}} \text{RNA} \xrightarrow{\text{reverse transcriptase}} \text{DNA}]$$

There are two opposing schools of thought about the way these many V genes are distributed in an animal. *Germline* theorists (Ref. 3.12) say that all antibody genes are present in the fertilized ovum and in every cell in the body. It is known that one antibody forming cell makes only one antibody (Chapter 4). According to the germline theory, this is because each cell selects only one from its complete repertoire of V genes for expression, just as other cells differentiate to a stage where they make hemoglobin only, or a particular hormone, while still possessing all other genes. All V genes are inherited through the germline DNA, and a conventional process of selective gene expression determines which cell makes which antibody.

The *somatic mutation* theory (Ref. 3.3) is quite different, and, at first sight, radical. Its proponents claim that there are relatively few (1–100) V genes at each Ig locus in the germline DNA. As the animal develops, all of those cells (lymphocytes) which will later be involved in antibody formation receive a copy of these few genes. Mutations occur in V genes, possibly at a higher rate than in other parts of the DNA, and special selective pressures encourage the mutants to survive (Chapter 8). The (human) individual ends up with perhaps 10^{12} antibody forming cells, each still with very few V genes, but now with 10^8 (a guess) different V genes in the population as a whole: the cells have diversified somatically. At all other loci the DNA may be essentially the same, regardless of what the cell is doing, but in the antibody V regions great variations occur from one cell to another.

An important new piece of information emerged as increasing numbers of V regions were sequenced. These polypeptide chains fall into *subgroups*. If 20 human V_κ sequences are aligned, all are seen to be different, but the differences are not random. They can be ordered into several groups, the members of any one differing by relatively few amino acids, while bigger differences exist between members of different groups. Figures 3.6 and 3.7 show some examples. These subgroups are not allotypic variants: every individual seems to have a large number of antibody V regions belonging to each subgroup. Such categories are found also within V_λ and V_H regions.

Some germline proponents were exultant when subgroups were discovered. This kind of pattern is similar to that found when one compares homologous proteins (e.g., cytochromes) from members of different species. Proteins from closely related species have similar sequences, and those from more distant

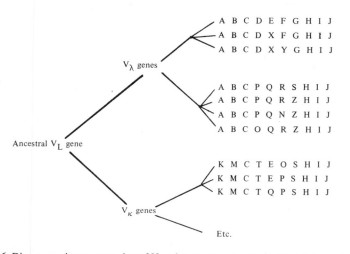

Fig. 3.6 Diagrammatic representation of V region sequences, showing how they can be arranged into a "tree." Letters are arbitrary representations of hypothetical amino acid sequences. Refer to Fig. 3.7 for actual examples.

species have sequences which reflect this difference. Clustering of similar amino acid sequences implies relatedness. Germline theorists argued that Ig subgroups showed how Ig V genes have evolved just like any other genes. Occasional mutations in a large inherited germline pool would produce the observed patterns over evolutionary time. An evolutionary tree could be drawn up (Fig. 3.6), similar to those constructed to show the evolution of other proteins.

Supporters of the somatic mutation theory retort that "they too can draw trees" (Cohn, Ref. 3.4). They envisage the same process of mutation and selection as their opponents, but enormously speeded up to occur within the lifespan of the individual. It is usually conceded that each subgroup represents one germline gene, since it is difficult to see how subgroups can be reproducibly created by a random process, but the terminal twigs of the tree, intrasubgroup variations, develop somatically, and are responsible for the vast bulk of immune diversity (further illustrated in Section 7.2).

This interesting controversy obviously cannot be solved without controlling the time dimension: a knowledge of any number of V region sequences at one point in time cannot discriminate between the two theories. We need to compare antibodies early in a response and later, for example, or to compare very young with older animals. We will return to this problem in Chapter 8. Amino acid variations between subgroups are about 40%, and within them about 20%. The differences between them are not always clear-cut, and more are being discovered all the time, i.e., further divisions are being found within existing sub-

Kappa Chains

	1	2	3	4	5	6	7	8	9	10	11	12	13	14	15	16	17	18	19	20
VκI Basic sequence	Asp	Ile	Gln	Met	Thr	Gln	Ser	Pro	Ser	Ser	Leu	Ser	Ala	Ser	Val	Gly	Asp	Arg	Val	Thr
Protein Ag																				
Roy																				
Eu									Thr											
Mon									Thr											
Bel				Leu																
Lux				Leu						Phe										
VκII Basic sequence	Glu	Ile	Val	Leu	Thr	Gln	Ser	Pro	Gly	Thr	Leu	Ser	Leu	Ser	Pro	Gly	Glu	Arg	Ala	Thr
Protein Nig	Lys																			
Rad																	Asp			
Cas																	Asp			
Smi									Ala											
Win	Asp								Ala											
VκIII Basic sequence	Asp	Ile	Val	Met	Thr	Gln	Ser	Pro	Leu	Ser	Leu	Pro	Val	Thr	Pro	Gly	Glu	Pro	Ala	Ser
Protein Tew																				
Mil				Leu																

Lambda Chains

	1	2	3	4	5	6	7	8	9	10	11	12	13	14	15	16	17	18	19	20
VλI Basic sequence	Glp	Ser	Val	Leu	Thr	Gln	Pro	Pro	GAP	Ser	Val	Ser	Gly	Ala	Pro	Gly	Gln	Arg	Val	Thr
Protein HS92																		Thr		
HS78				Ala																
HBJ7											Ala			Thr				Gly		
HBJ11											Ala			Thr						
VλII Basic sequence	Glp	Ser	Ala	Leu	Thr	Gln	Pro	Ala	GAP	Ser	Val	Ser	Gly	Ser	Pro	Gly	Gln	Ser	Ile	Thr
Protein HS68																				
HBJ8							Ala													
HS86				Pro			Ala										Glu			
VλIII Basic sequence		Tyr	Val	Leu	Thr	Gln	Pro	Pro	GAP	Ser	Val	Ser	Val	Ser	Pro	Gly	Gln	Thr	Ala	Ser
Protein Kern		Ala																		Val
X		Asp																		

	1	2	3	4	5	6	7	8	9	10	11	12	13	14	15	16	17	18	19	20
VλIV Basic sequence	Glp	Ser	Ala	Leu	Thr	Gln	Pro	Pro	GAP	Ser	Ala	Ser	Gly	Ser	Pro	Gly	Gln	Ser	Val	Thr
Protein Bo																				
HBJ2																				
VλV Basic sequence		Ser	Glu	Leu	Thr	Gln	Asp	Pro	GAP	Ala	Val	Ser	Val	Ala	Leu	Gly	Gln	Thr	Val	Arg
Protein Sh																				

Heavy Chains

	1	2	3	4	5	6	7	8	9	10	11	12	13	14	15	16	17	18	19	20
VHI Basic sequence	Glp	Val	Gln	Leu	Val	Glu	Ser	Gly	GAP	Ala	Glu	Val	Lys	Lys	Pro	Gly	Ala	Ser	Val	Lys
Protein Eu γ1							Gln										Ser			
Ste γ1			His								Ser								Met	
Ca γ1							Gln								Arg					
Zuc γ3 HCD[a]					Val						Asp	Leu	Val				Gly			
VHH Basic sequence	Glp	Val	Thr	Leu	Arg	Glu	Ser	Gly	GAP	Pro	Ala	Leu	Val	Lys	Pro	Thr	Gln	Thr	Leu	Thr
Protein Daw γ1															Arg					
Cor γ1																				
Ou μ							Thr										Lys		Pro	
He γ1						Lys		Asn					Thr							
VHIII Basic sequence	Glu	Val	Gln	Leu	Val	Glu	Ser	Gly	GAP	Gly	Gly	Leu	Val	Glu	Pro	Gly	Gly	Ser	Leu	Arg
Vin γ4														Ile						
Hiγ HCD[a]	Gly		Leu									Val	Ser	Ile		?				
Wat γ2																				
For α1			Ile													Lys	Gly			
Low α2																?				
Jor α1	Glx		Glx				Glx									Glx				
Ha α																Gly				
Wo μ																				
Til μ and γ						Leu														
Sha					Met								Val		Lys					
Wei γ	Asx		Glx		Met	Glx							Ala		Lys			Glx		
VHIV Basic sequence	Glp	Ser	Val	Leu	Asx															
Dos μ			Ala																	
Dau μ																				
Bus μ																				
Bal μ				Ala																
Re μ			Ala																	

Fig. 3.7 Subgroups of variable regions of κ, λ, and heavy chains. Nomenclature is that recommended by the World Health Organization. Light chain sequence data are here selected to show the presence of further divisions of each basic sequence (see text). Solid lines indicate identity to basic sequence of corresponding subgroup. Glp indicates pyrrolidonecarboxylic acid; Glx indicates glutamic acid or glutamine. Gaps have been arbitrarily inserted in λ and heavy chains to show their evolutionary relationship to each other and to κ chains. (From Fudenberg et al. Ref. 3.9.)

groups. Nevertheless, the present conventional view is that if somatic mutation is responsible for diversity, then it operates on an initial number of V genes which is approximately equal to the number of subgroups currently identified. This gives rise to the "complete" table of human germline Ig genes shown in Table 3.2. Most somatic mutationalists would probably want to say that there may be more than one V gene inherited per subgroup. Current research is identifying increasing numbers of certain defined antibody specificities which seem to be inherited as germline V genes (Ref. 3.8).

Under the general heading of "somatic mutation" we should mention also that a number of mechanisms have been proposed in which recombination between a small initial array of V genes creates many more. The most interesting of these is the idea that small stretches of DNA might be inserted into larger framework genes (Wu and Kabat). There is evidence that identical hypervariable regions can turn up within quite different V gene backgrounds. One of the most striking recent examples (Capra) concerns two IgM human proteins (from different donors): one had a $V_\kappa I$ L chain, and the other a $V_\kappa III$, yet two of the three hypervariable regions in these very different L chains were identical.

3.7 MOLECULAR HYBRIDIZATION

While amino acid sequence studies have not conclusively shown whether few or many V genes are inherited, the last few years have seen the application of a technique which may finally answer the question by directly counting the number of genes in a cell's DNA. This is molecular hybridization (Ref. 3.5).

Moderately pure, homogeneous mRNA may be extracted from myeloma cells. This is radiolabeled and hybridized with a vast excess of genome DNA from various tissues. [Alternatively a radioactive complementary DNA (cDNA) may be prepared with reverse transcriptase.] The rate of hybridization depends on the number of complementary gene copies in the DNA: if there are many, union will be rapid. This procedure is technically complex; unambiguous interpretation of the results depends on knowing the purity of the mRNA and the degree of complementarity necessary for annealing under particular experimental conditions. Several groups of workers in this area have, however, agreed that V region subgroups each contain very few genes (one to three), which, if true, appears to prove the somatic generation of V gene diversity.

3.8 EVOLUTION OF Ig GENES

Crystallographic and amino acid sequence studies have shown that each Ig polypeptide is folded into a series of compact globular *domains* (Edelman), each

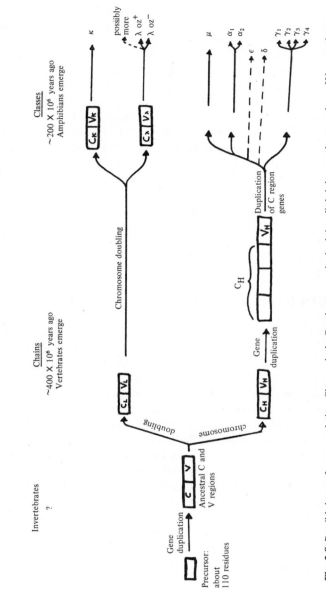

Fig. 3.8 Possible human Ig gene evolution. Changes in the C region are emphasized since little is known about numbers of V genes: these may also have undergone amplification in numbers. The crude time scale is located on the assumption that rates of mutation in C genes have been approximately constant throughout evolution. (Adapted from Fudenberg *et al.*, Ref. 3.9.)

stabilized by internal disulfide bonds (Fig. 3.5). Each domain is about the size of a V region. Thus a light chain has two domains, $V_L + C_L$, while a γ chain has four, as shown in Fig. 3.5 (a μ chain has five). The C_H region domains show considerable sequence homology (30–40%) with each other and with C_L. Homology between V and C domains is much less obvious, but the two are similar in size.

It appears likely that the domains are the unit of Ig evolution and that the first Ig gene may have been one coding for a polypeptide about the size of the modern V region, 110 amino acids (Fig. 3.8). This was probably present at a prevertebrate era of evolution. By gene duplication, it doubled in length, making a primitive, linked VC combination. The V/C divergence probably occurred very early since the V and C regions of modern Ig polypeptides show very little homology. Doubling of the chromosomes or of large regions of DNA at about the stage of vertebrate emergence could have generated separate H and L loci. (Both single and multiple gene duplications are thought to have occurred in the evolution of other polymorphic proteins.) The ancestral L region duplicated again, making κ and λ loci, while the H region may have reduplicated in a more complex way, forming the longer C_H chains which, however, retain some internal evidence of their origin from small subunits. Subclasses, judging by their greater similarities, diverged late. This evolution seems fairly clear for the C regions: for V regions, little is known, but if subgroups reflect different germline genes, they must also have reduplicated. If the germline theory is correct, reduplication of V regions must have been very extensive.

3.9 SUMMARY

1. Most immunoglobulin molecules consist of two identical light chains (κ or λ), and two identical heavy chains. The two kinds of L chains, and H chains are coded for at three separate, unlinked genetic loci. The chains are synthesized separately and combined (by disulfide bridges) in the cytoplasm to make whole antibody molecules.

2. Each Ig polypeptide has two regions, V (variable) and C (constant), coded for by separate genes. The two sets of genes are closely linked. It is probable that translocation at the DNA level brings about juxtaposition of a V and C gene so that they can be read off as a single RNA message. Thus two genes give one Ig polypeptide chain.

3. Multiple C genes exist at each Ig locus in every individual, e.g., there are nine known H chain genes in humans coding for different isotypes (i.e., five classes and subclasses): γ_1, γ_2, γ_3, γ_4, α_1, α_2, μ, δ, and ϵ. Ig's with different H chain classes have different biological properties.

48   3. Molecular Biology of Antibody Formation

4. The number of V genes at each locus is debatable. Many thousands of V regions must exist in each individual. Germline theorists say these are all represented in the germline by genes at one of the three loci, while proponents of somatic mutation say there is only one or very few for each V region subgroup (these subgroups are groups of V sequences with greater than average similarities). It is probable that any V gene at one locus can combine with any C gene at the same locus to allow transcription of a complete message.

FURTHER READING

3.1   Amzel, L. M., Poljak, R. J., Saul, F., Varga, J. M., and Richards, F. F. (1974). The three dimensional structure of a combining region-ligand complex of immunoglobulin NEW at 3.5-Å resolution. *Proc. Natl. Acad. Sci. (U.S.A.)* **71**, 1427.
3.2   Bevan, M. J., Parkhouse, R. M. E., Williamson, A. R., and Askonas, B. A. (1972). Biosynthesis of immunoglobulins. *Prog. Biophys. Mol. Biol.* **25**, 131.
3.3   Cohn, M. (1970). Selection under a somatic model. *Cell. Immunol.* **1**, 461.
3.4   Cohn, M. (1974). "A rationale for ordering the data on antibody diversification". *In* "Progress in Immunology" (L. Brent and J. Holborow, eds.), Vol. II, p. 261. North Holland, Amsterdam.
3.5   Cunningham, A. J. (ed.). (1976). "The Generation of Antibody Diversity: A New Look." Academic Press, London. Contains a number of papers by workers in this field, including two on molecular hybridization.
3.6   Edelman, G. M. (1973). Antibody structure and molecular biology (Nobel lecture). *Science* **180**, 830.
3.7   Edelman, G. M., Cunningham, B. A., Gall, W. E., Gottlieb, P. D., Rutishauser, U., and Waxdal, M. J. (1969). The covalent structure of an entire γ G immunoglobulin molecule. *Proc. Natl. Acad. Sci. (U.S.A.)* **63**, 78.
3.8   Eichmann, K. (1975). Genetic control of antibody specificity in the mouse. *Immunogenetics* **2**, 491.
3.9   Fudenberg, H. H., Pink, J. R. L., Stites, D. P., and An-Chuang Wang (1972). "Basic Immunogenetics." Oxford Univ. Press, London.
3.10 Gally, J. A. and Edelman, G. M. (1972). The genetic control of immunoglobulin synthesis. *Annu. Rev. Genet.* **6**, 1.
3.11 Hildemann, W. H. (1970). "Immunogenetics." Holden-Day, San Francisco, California.
3.12 Hood, L. and Prahl, J. (1971). The immune system: a model for differentiation in higher organisms. *Adv. Immunol.* **14**, 291.
3.13 Milstein, C. and Pink, J. R. L. (1970). Structure and evolution of immunoglobulins. *Prog. Biophys. Mol. Biol.* **21**, 209.
3.14 Natvig, J. B. and Kunkel, H. G. (1973). Human immunoglobulins: classes, subclasses, genetic variants and idiotypes. *Adv. Immunol.* **16**, 1.
3.15 Poljak R. J. (1975). X-ray diffraction studies of immunoglobulins. *Adv. Immunol.* **21**, 1.
3.16 Porter, R. R. (1973). Structural studies of immunoglobulins (Nobel lecture). *Science* **180**, 713.
3.17 Williamson, A. R. (1976). The biological origin of antibody diversity. *Annu. Rev. Biochem.* **45**, 467. A concise recent review of Ig structure, genetics, and molecular hybridization.

QUESTIONS

3.1 How might you distinguish, by examining serum, between (a) a clinical condition in which there was overproduction of all globulins; (b) a patient bearing a myeloma?

3.2 How would you measure the half-life of IgG molecules in the serum of a mouse (i.e., within the living animal)?

3.3 Given a mixture of IgM and IgG antibodies with equal affinities for the same antigenic determinant, which is likely to bind most firmly to a large antigen molecule with many of these determinants, and why?

Lymphocytes, Lymphoid Tissue, and Antibody Forming Cells

4.1 THE SINGLE CELL AS THE UNIT IN IMMUNOLOGY

Any biological phenomenon can be explained at many different levels, ranging from its molecular and genetic basis through to cellular and tissue events, and to effects in the whole animal. Different disciplines tend to have characteristic levels of study. For example, explanations of cellular metabolism are often sought in terms of the behavior of small molecules; viral replication is described in the language of proteins and nucleic acids; gross anatomy, by contrast, deals with organs and their relations to one other—any explanation in terms of DNA would be pointless. For immunology, a fairly wide range of levels of study is important, certainly including the genetic and the molecular, but most current research in the subject centers around the lymphoid *cell* as a unit. Many of the ruling theories are framed in terms of cells rather than molecules. This is because most of the events occurring within cells, the biosynthesis of protein, for example, are essentially the same in the cells of the immune system as in other kinds. The characteristic phenomena of the subject are to be found in the way immune cells are diversified and react with one another and with their environment. (The question of choosing appropriate levels of study within a particular discipline like immunology is discussed more fully in Ref. 4.3.)

In the next three chapters we will study the cells which constitute the immune system. Then, equipped with this information, and with the knowledge of antibody reactions and structure discussed in Chapters 2 and 3, we can approach the central problem in the subject: how does an individual develop a repertoire of specificities without reacting against itself?

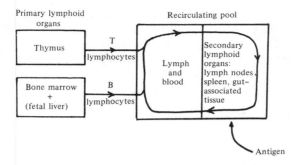

Fig. 4.1 Production and recirculation of T and B lymphocytes.

4.2 LYMPHOID TISSUE

The most important cells in the immune system are *lymphocytes* (literally "lymph cells"). *Lymphoid tissue* is a term which includes these cells, together with the *primary* or *central* lymphoid organs where they are produced (thymus and bone marrow in adult mammals), and the *secondary* or *peripheral* lymphoid organs where lymphocytes come into contact with antigen and make immune responses (Fig. 4.1). The most important of the peripheral organs are *lymph nodes* (below), and parts of the spleen. There is also organized lymphoid tissue associated with the gut: the tonsils, the appendix, and Peyer's patches, these last being nodules in the wall of the intestine.

4.2.1 Lymphocytes

Small lymphocytes are spherical cells, about 6 μm in diameter in most species. They are relatively inactive metabolically, i.e., do not divide, and have condensed chromatin in a nucleus which leaves little room for a thin shell of rather featureless cytoplasm. Their most obvious property is that they are continuously circulating around the body. Upon appropriate stimulation with antigens, small lymphocytes *transform* (i.e., change without dividing) into much larger cells (up to about 15 μm in diameter) which can divide, and have many more cytoplasmic ribosomes and mitochondria as evidence of their greater metabolic activity (Section 4.9). The nomenclature and interrelationships of these more active cells are complex, but they include "medium" and "large" lymphocytes (Fig. 4.2). Small lymphocytes are, however, the predominant recirculating type.

The function of small lymphocytes was unknown until surprisingly recently. Around 1960 Gowans showed that the majority of lymphocytes in a rat could be drained out through a fine tube or cannula inserted into the thoracic lymph duct

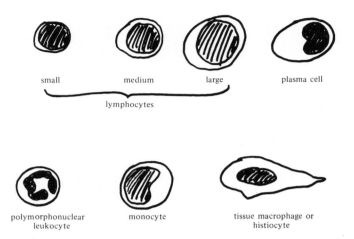

Fig. 4.2 Diagram of the main kinds of cells involved in reactions to foreign material. Lymphocytes and plasma cells are the effectors of specific immune reactions. Polymorphs and macrophages act as nonspecific scavenger cells (although macrophages may also adsorb antibody and take part in specific immune reactions). A small lymphocyte, spread on a slide, is about $7\mu m$ in diameter. Photographs of these cells can be found in textbooks of hematology, among which that of Bessis (Ref. 4.1) is a beautiful and modern example.

(see below) and left in place for several days. Such lymphocyte-depleted animals had a greatly decreased ability to respond immunologically. Their powers could be restored by injecting lymphocytes collected from the thoracic duct of another rat. Only the small lymphocytes (and not the small proportion of circulating larger ones) were necessary for this restoration: thus these cells were identified as essential for immune responses (Fig. 4.3).

4.2.2 Differentiation of T and B Lymphocytes

It has become clear in the last few years that lymphocytes fall into two major categories, called T and B (Ref. 4.5). These have quite different functions: B lymphocytes become antibody forming cells, while T lymphocytes develop into cells responsible for "cell-mediated" immune reactions (Chapter 9) and for regulating immune responses. Their detailed properties will be discussed later, but for the present it is helpful to consider briefly how this separation into two classes is accomplished during development.

The yolk sac and, later, the fetal liver of mammalian embryos contain *stem* cells whose offspring can become any of several kinds of hemopoietic (blood forming) cell: erythrocytes, granulocytes, (Section 4.2.4), megakaryocytes (platelet producers), or lymphocytes (Fig. 4.4). In adult animals, stem cells are

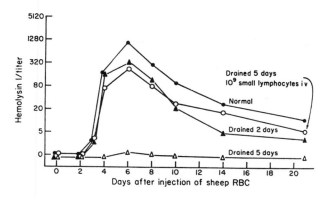

Fig. 4.3 Hemolysin response to a single intravenous injection of 10^8 sheep erythrocytes in normal rats and in lymphocyte-depleted rats injected intravenously with small lymphocytes. ●———●, the mean response of fourteen normal rats; ▲———▲, the mean response of 4 rats after drainage from a thoracic duct fistula for 2 days; △———△, the mean response of ten rats after 5 day's drainage. ○———○, the mean response of four rats depleted of lymphocytes for 5 days and then injected with 10^9 small lymphocytes (from McGregor and Gowans, Ref. 4.6).

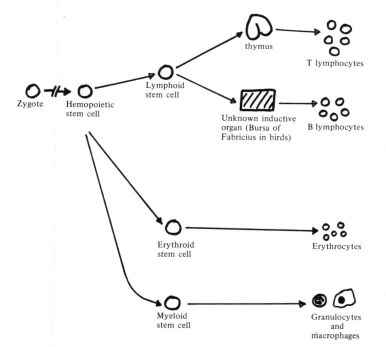

Fig. 4.4 The development of T and B lymphocytes, and their relationship to other cells of the blood. The "lymphoid stem cell" is hypothetical; erythroid and myeloid stem cells can be experimentally distinguished from their common ancestor.

produced in bone marrow. The subsequent fate of a particular stem cell probably depends on the inductive environment into which it migrates. A hemopoietic stem cell (or its immediate descendants), after migrating into the thymus, will divide repeatedly, giving small lymphocytes of the T type. Whether there is a corresponding inductive organ for B cells in mammals is not known (birds do have an inductive organ for B cells corresponding to the thymus; this is the bursa of Fabricius, a cloacal lymphoid organ). The initials T and B come from the organs involved in directing primitive lymphoid cells along either pathway. In the case of B cells, it is convenient that although mammals have no bursa, they do manufacture B cells in their bone marrow. The development of these cells is discussed further in Ref 4.7 and in Section 5.2.5.

T and B lymphocytes look the same when examined by light or electron microscopy. An early report that under the scanning electron microscope B cells had more surface projections than T cells appears now to have been incorrect.

4.2.3 The Lymphatic Circulation

The lymphatic system of the body collects fluid or lymph which diffuses from capillary blood vessels into the surrounding tissues. This fluid is returned to the blood via a system of delicate thin-walled vessels. On the way back to the blood, the lymph in any part of the body passes through a chain of *lymph nodes,* small glandular filters, one of whose functions is to intercept foreign substances which enter the tissues and to stop them from reaching the blood (Fig. 4.5). The lymphocytes themselves do not reach the extracellular tissue fluids in large numbers. Instead, they escape from the blood while it is passing through lymph nodes, making their exit through the walls of postcapillary venules (Fig. 4.6). Once in the node they are swept along with the lymph into efferent lymphatic vessels which flow into the next node of a chain. After several nodes, the lymph with its passenger lymphocytes drains into common large ducts (the thoracic and cervical lymph ducts) which in turn discharge into the large veins near the heart.

This recirculation of cells is continuous and fairly rapid. Work with sheep has shown that of the lymphocytes in the blood passing through a peripheral node, about 10% escape into the lymph (Fig. 4.6). Mice have a total of about 2×10^8 lymphocytes in their recirculating pool: 1–2% of these per hour enter the blood from the thoracic duct. Both T and B cells recirculate, although T cells do so more efficiently: about 80–85% of thoracic duct lymphocytes (in mice) are T cells. New B cells which have recently come from the bone marrow tend to localize in the spleen. Memory cells of both T and B lines, that is, lymphocytes which have been generated as a result of contact with antigen (Chapter 6), seem to recirculate continuously, and have been shown to live for months or even years without dividing. References 4.4 and 4.10 contain more information about the lymphatic system and lymphocyte recirculation.

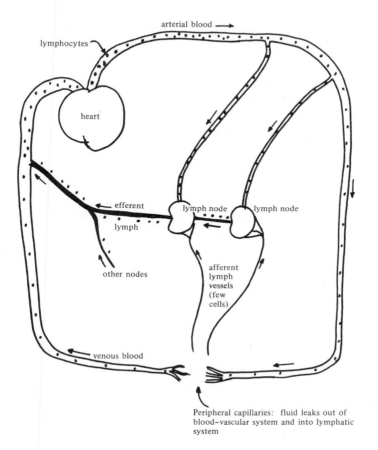

arterial blood ⟶

lymphocytes

heart

efferent

lymph

lymph node   lymph node

other nodes

afferent
lymph
vessels
(few
cells)

venous blood

Peripheral capillaries: fluid leaks out of
blood–vascular system and into lymphatic
system

Fig. 4.5 Blood and lymphatic circulations. Many lymphocytes continually recirculate from blood
to lymph, escaping from the blood within lymph nodes.

4.2.4 Phagocytic cells

Metazoan animals, from the most phylogentically primitive upward, have
specialized cells which *phagocytize* (eat) foreign particles. Vertebrate *phagocytes*
fall into two groups, both derived from the same hemopoietic stem cells (Fig.
4.4). The polymorphonuclear leukocytes or granulocytes are short-lived cells
found in blood, which have, as their name implies, lobed nuclei and large
cytoplasmic granules (Fig. 4.2). Mononuclear phagocytes have round nuclei;
they are produced in the bone marrow, occur as spherical monocytes in blood,
and develop into irregularly shaped fixed (noncirculating) *macrophages,* resident

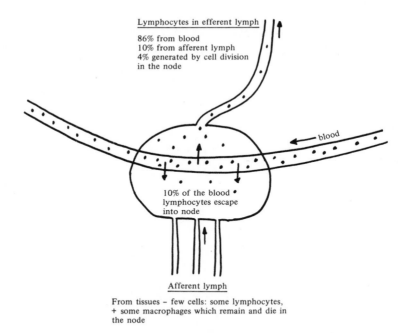

Lymphocytes in efferent lymph

86% from blood
10% from afferent lymph
4% generated by cell division
in the node

blood

10% of the blood
lymphocytes escape
into node

Afferent lymph

From tissues – few cells: some lymphocytes,
+ some macrophages which remain and die in
the node

Fig. 4.6 Lymphocyte traffic in a peripheral node. The efferent lymph contains lymphocytes most of which have come from the blood via postcapillary venules. The number of lymphocytes passing into the lymph, and the proportion in efferent lymph which have arisen by division within the node, are both greatly increased by antigenic stimulation. Note that the *afferent* lymph of nodes higher up a chain will receive all of the cells from the *efferent* lymph of a more peripheral node.

in lymphoid tissue and in other sites such as liver sinusoids, pulmonary alveoli, and the peritoneal cavity. The "reticuloendothelial system" or "mononuclear phagocytic system" are names sometimes used to embrace the functionally similar group of scattered phagocytic mononuclear cells throughout the body. An important property of macrophages and polymorphs is that IgG antibody adheres to them via its Fc part. Such antibody is said to be *cytophilic* (cell-loving), and its attachment implies that the cells have a receptor for γ chain Fc piece.

A sharp distinction must be drawn between lymphocytes, on the one hand, and the phagocytic polymorphs, monocytes, and macrophages, on the other. Lymphocytes are *specific* cells, that is, any one lymphocyte will take part in only one particular immune reaction (for reasons which will become clearer in the next chapter). The phagocytes are nonspecific cells, each of which can ingest a variety of foreign particles. Those which circulate around the body (polymorphs and monocytes) do so only in the blood, and are rarely found in the lymph.

4.3 LOCAL ANTIGENIC STIMULATION

We can now outline the events which follow a local bacterial infection in the body. There is, first, an inflammatory response, a useful but (phylogenetically) primitive reaction involving increased blood flow to the area, the extravasation (escape from the blood) within minutes of polymorphs, which phagocytize bacteria, and the later appearance of macrophages which digest both bacteria and dead polymorphs. (Stimulation with nonliving antigens usually provokes less inflammation and polymorph accumulation.) Much slower to develop (over a period of days, rather than hours), is the immune reaction. Antigen, either whole bacteria or their products, reaches the local lymph node (Fig. 4.7) where some is trapped by macrophages lining subcapsular and medullary sinuses, while some appears on the outer surface of "dendritic" (branching) processes of macrophages in the cortical follicles (the localization of antigen is thoroughly dis-

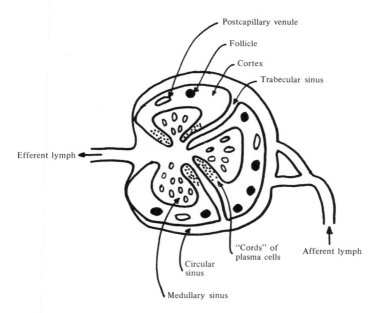

Postcapillary venule

Follicle

Cortex

Trabecular sinus

Efferent lymph

"Cords" of plasma cells

Afferent lymph

Circular sinus

Medullary sinus

Fig. 4.7 Diagram of a lymph node (after Nossal, Ref. 1.4). Lymph enters the node from the tissues or from a node lower in the chain and filters through to the medullary sinuses. Some antigen is taken up by macrophages here, and some is trapped in the outer cortical region. Lymphocytes enter the node from the blood through postcapillary venules in the cortex. The follicles are dense nodules of lymphocytes which may show a lot of mitotic activity after antigenic stimulation of the node. Most antibody is produced by stimulated lymphocytes which migrate from the cortex into the medullary cords where many of them turn into plasma cells (see also Ref. 4.8).

cussed in Ref. 4.8). Circulating lymphocytes make contact with antigen-bearing macrophages, and some of these lymphocytes are stimulated to turn into antibody forming cells, which typically stay in the node; there is little point in their recirculating further since it is now their product, antibody, which is useful to the animal, as it reacts with the antigen in the initial infected area or in the blood.

Antibody formation requires cooperative events between T cells, B cells, and macrophages (Chapter 5). The detailed physiology of these cellular interactions in stimulated nodes is complex and still poorly understood, but we can add some detail to the outline given above. Rather surprisingly (given the need for cell interaction), lymphoid tissue has distinct T- or B- "dependent" areas. The cortical region of a node (except for follicles) is T-dependent, i.e., it is depleted of lymphocytes by procedures which remove T cells rather than B from the body (draining the thoracic duct, antilymphocyte serum, neonatal thymectomy, and genetic absence of a thymus, explained in Chapter 5). The follicles and medullary regions (Fig. 4.7), by contrast, contain mainly B cells. Within 24 hours of antigenic stimulation, proliferation and "blast" formation (enlargement) of T cells occurs in the cortex. Many of these activated T cells escape to the circulating pool. The follicles expand, but more slowly. They are nodules which have a "germinal center" comprising large lymphoid cells and macrophages, surrounded by B cells that proliferate after antigen stimulation. It seems probable that these B cells migrate to the medullary cords (Fig. 4.7) where most of the actual antibody formation takes place. Small numbers of T cells have also been detected within stimulated follicles. A proportion of recently activated T and B cells migrate, for unknown reasons, to the lamina propia (connective tissue under the mucosal epithelium) and Peyer's patches of the gut.

Immune responses may often be increased by injecting antigen mixed with *adjuvants* (from the *Latin* "adjuvare," to help), agents which cause increased local recirculation of lymphocytes, and slow, continual release of antigen from a "depot" in an area of localized inflammation. *Freund's complete adjuvant* is commonly used. It consists of an emulsion of mineral oil, detergent, and mycobacteria into which antigen is incorporated.

The overall "logic" of antigen–lymphocyte interactions is fairly clear. Foreign antigens are carried to specialized lymphoid tissue. If these antigens enter the body via the skin or gut wall they go to local "draining" nodes; if they reach the blood they are more likely to end up in the periarteriolar lymphatic sheaths of the spleen, which behave like nodes. Small lymphocytes recirculate through these areas, and since each cell can react with few antigens (Chapter 5) the purpose of this traffic must be to bring the "right" lymphocytes and antigen together. The organized lymphoid tissue then provides a suitable microenvironment for the complex interaction necessary to goad lymphocytes into antibody formation or other activities.

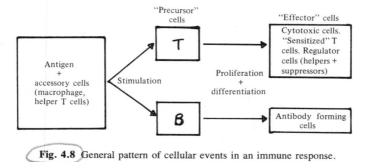

Fig. 4.8 General pattern of cellular events in an immune response.

4.4 GENERAL PATTERN OF CELLULAR EVENTS IN AN IMMUNE RESPONSE

As Fig. 4.8 shows in outline, the stimulation of either T or B cells by antigen involves grossly similar processes. Since events in the B line are much better understood we will look at them first and in most detail, working backward from the identification of antibody forming cells (see Section 4.5) to the complexities of their induction (see Chapter 5).

4.5 METHODS FOR DETECTING SINGLE ANTIBODY FORMING CELLS

Lymphoid tissue was recognized early as a major site of antibody production, since antibody appeared in high concentration in lymph nodes draining the site of injection of antigen, and the lymph coming from these nodes had a higher antibody titer than blood. For many years there was fierce argument about which cells actually produced the antibody: some workers thought it was lymphocytes, because these were the main type found in lymph nodes; others thought plasma cells (Section 4.6.1), because these cells began to appear in large numbers when antibody was being synthesized.

4.5.1 Immunofluorescence

The first direct method for demonstrating immunoglobulin containing cells was the fluorescent antibody technique, introduced by Coons in 1942. A fluorescent dye, e.g., fluorescein or rhodamine, is chemically coupled to specific antibody. The antibody is then allowed to react with histological sections of a tissue. The antigens against which the antibody is directed will show up as brightly

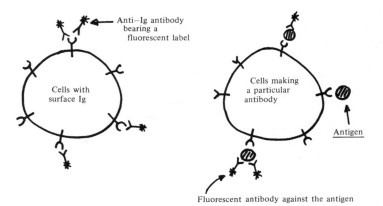

Fig. 4.9 Fluorescent antibody technique for detecting Ig, or specific antibody forming cells.

fluorescent areas (Fig. 4.9). If cells containing Ig are to be detected, the fluorescent dye is coupled to an anti-Ig antibody. To find those cells (in a tissue or population) able to react with a particular antigen, the "sandwich" variation of the technique is used. The tissue is first pretreated with antigen, which binds firmly to the specifically reactive cells. Fluorescent-labeled antibody against the same antigen is then added (Fig. 4.9). Immunofluorescence is a technique which can detect a wide variety of cellular and tissue antigens. It is extensively used in medical diagnosis and in research in many biological fields.

4.5.2 Micromanipulative Techniques

A cell suspension is made from lymphoid tissue which is undergoing an immune response. (For example, the popliteal node might be taken from a mouse injected several days earlier in the hind footpad with *Salmonella* organisms.) These cells may be handled individually with a micromanipulator to which a very fine pipette is attached (Fig. 4.10). If single cells are incubated in microdroplets of a suitable culture medium, then each droplet can be tested for the presence or absence of specific antibody. In the early work of Nossal, the test was to put into each drop a number of motile *Salmonella,* which were immobilized if antibody to their flagella had been produced. Other antigens have been used. For example, bacteriophage neutralization may be measured on this very small scale, or the lysis or red blood cells by instilling them, together with complement, into droplets containing lymphoid cells from animals immunized with the same red blood cell antigen. This kind of work is rather tedious but does provide unequivocal information on the properties of antibody forming cells. For example, it can tell us how many different antibodies are produced by one cell (Section 4.6.2).

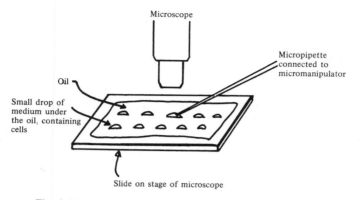

Fig. 4.10 Micromanipulation. (See Ref. 4.2 for further details.)

4.5.3 The Hemolytic Plaque Technique (Jerne and Ingraham)

This is one of the most important techniques developed in immunology during the last few years. A variant of the original method is described here. Lymphoid cells from an animal immunized with erythrocytes from other species are mixed in a tube with complement (Section 2.2.6) and with more erythrocytes of the type used for immunization. The contents of the tube are then pipetted into a very shallow chamber formed by sticking together two microscope slides. This is sealed, and incubated for 1 hour at 37°C, being kept in a horizontal position. Cells settle to the bottom surface. Antibody, released by the small proportion of active cells, attaches to the surrounding erythrocytes which are lysed by complement, leaving a small plaque about 0.5 mm in diameter (Fig. 4.11). This test can be modified to detect cells producing antibody against a variety of antigens by coupling the antigen to the target red cell (Fig. 4.11).

The plaque test can also distinguish cells producing antibody of different Ig classes. Cells releasing IgM antibody are the only ones which will form plaques directly, as described above, and a single molecule of IgM is apparently sufficient to activate a local complement cascade and punch a hole in the erythrocyte membrane (Section 2.2.6). Cells making IgG antibody do not produce plaques unless a "developing" serum is added. This consists of anti-antibody, that is, antibody against Ig. Rabbit antibody against mouse IgG is often used to develop mouse IgG plaques. It appears that IgG antibody on a membrane will not activate complement unless two molecules are attached close together. The anti-antibody can, however, increase the size of the Ig complex attached to the red cell (Fig. 4.12) so that it will fix complement.

The great feature of the plaque technique, apart from its simplicity, is its

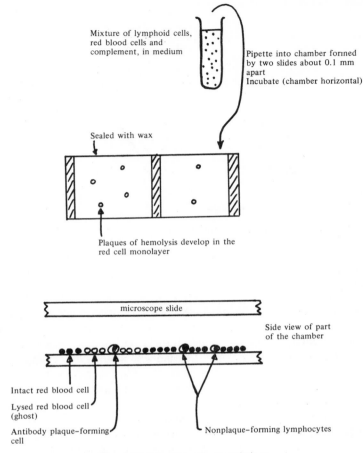

Mixture of lymphoid cells, red blood cells and complement, in medium

Pipette into chamber formed by two slides about 0.1 mm apart
Incubate (chamber horizontal)

Sealed with wax

Plaques of hemolysis develop in the red cell monolayer

microscope slide

Side view of part of the chamber

Intact red blood cell

Lysed red blood cell (ghost)

Antibody plaque-forming cell

Nonplaque-forming lymphocytes

Fig. 4.11 Hemolytic plaque technique.

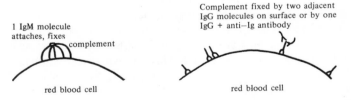

1 IgM molecule attaches, fixes
complement

red blood cell

Complement fixed by two adjacent IgG molecules on surface or by one IgG + anti-Ig antibody

red blood cell

Fig. 4.12 Lysis of red blood cells by antibody and complement. A single molecule of IgM antibody is thought to be enough to fix complement and lyse a red cell. The smaller IgG molecules will not do so, unless two of them attach to the red cell surface close together. But a single IgG molecule may be made "bigger" by combination with anti-Ig molecules, producing a complex which will now fix complement.

power to detect a single antibody forming cell among a vast excess (10^7) of inactive cells. Thus it can be much more sensitive than a serum antibody titration. It provides information on the number of antibody forming cells present in a particular piece of lymphoid tissue at a given time. Serum titers, on the other hand, represent the cumulative product of many scattered lymphoid cells.

4.6 PROPERTIES OF THE ANTIBODY FORMING CELL

4.6.1 Morphology

The best evidence comes from immunofluorescence and from micromanipulative work in which single cells were studied by light microscopy, or sectioned and examined in the electron microscope. A wide variety of lymphoid mononuclear cells have been found to produce antibody. The most differentiated type is the *plasma* cell, which, under the electron microscope, has a cytoplasm filled with polyribosomes and channels of endoplasmic reticulum. This kind of morphology is characteristic of many kinds of protein exporting cell. However, other cells with less organized cytoplasm are also commonly identified as antibody formers: "blasts" are very large cells (15 μm or more in diameter) with little cytoplasm and an enormous nucleus that shows a fine fibrillary chromatin pattern; somewhat smaller cells with relatively more cytoplasm are usually called "immature plasma cells" in the belief that they are destined to generate plasma cell progeny; occasional antibody forming cells look like small lymphocytes. All of these cells have a cytoplasm which is "basophilic," i.e., stains dark blue with Leishman's or related stains, indicating the presence of cytoplasmic RNA. Photographs can be inspected in Ref. 4.1.

4.6.2 A Single Cell Produces Antibody of Only One Specificity

This discovery, of central importance to immunological theory (Chapter 7), was made using micromanipulative techniques. Lymph nodes were taken from an animal immunized simultaneously with two species of *Salmonella,* and individual cells were tested in microdrops against a combination of both antigens. It was found (Nossal, Ref. 4.9) that virtually all cells which immobilized one species of bacteria did not affect the other.

This may be demonstrated more easily using the hemolytic plaque technique. A mouse is immunized simultaneously with two non-cross-reacting erythrocyte types (e.g., sheep and horse), and its lymphoid cells (e.g., from spleen) tested for antibody formation as described in Section 4.5.3, but using a mixed indicator layer containing equal numbers of both red cell types. The resulting plaques are now not clear but "cloudy" or partial, and under the microscope it can be seen that within a plaque, either the sheep or the horse red cells, but not both, are lysed.

4.6.3 A Single Cell Produces Antibody of Only One Class

Experiments where antibody-forming cells were stained simultaneously with anti-μ and anti-γ antibody, each coupled to a different fluorescent dye, have shown that each cell usually produces antibody of only one class. This has been confirmed by some rather complex experiments using the hemolytic plaque technique, e.g., individual cells were first allowed to make IgM antibody, then the same cells were micromanipulated into fresh medium and tested, in the presence of sufficiently concentrated anti-μ serum to inhibit direct plaques, for their ability to make indirect (IgG) plaques. Each cell also secretes only one kind of L chain. However, a small proportion of cells containing both IgM and IgG is sometimes found. Furthermore, the injection of mice early in life with large amounts of anti-μ antibody may prevent subsequent production of IgG and IgA immunoglobulins. Thus it seems probable that as antibody forming cells proliferate, a switch from μ to γ or α chain production commonly occurs within the same cell at some stage in the development of a clone (Section 4.9). The properties of antibody-forming cells are more fully explored in Ref. 4.2.

4.7 KINETICS OF APPEARANCE OF ANTIBODY FORMING CELLS IN LYMPHOID TISSUE

In a typical experiment to study the cellular basis of antibody formation a group of mice are immunized with sheep erythrocytes in one hind footpad, and popliteal nodes removed at intervals and assayed for plaque forming cells using the hemolytic plaque technique (Fig. 4.13). No active cells at all can be found during the first 2–3 days. Then IgM plaques appear very rapidly, reaching peak numbers at days 4–5 when about one cell in every 500 in the node is producing specific antibody. This rapid increase is a result of two processes:

1. The "recruitment" of new lymphocytes from the circulating pool, to take part in the specific immune response.

2. The proliferation of stimulated cells, so that each gives rise to a number of progeny. At about 6 days, the first IgG plaque formers are seen, and these are the predominant type after this time. Numbers of antibody forming cells then gradually decline, although there are still a few present 1–2 months later. Serum antibody levels follow plaque kinetics, as would be expected, but they decline more slowly, since (IgG) antibody has a half-life (Table 3.1) of about 3 weeks.

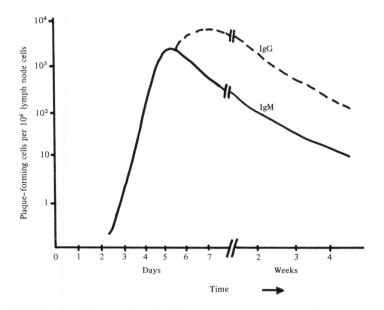

Fig. 4.13 Kinetics of the plaque forming cell response in a mouse popliteal lymph node stimulated with sheep erythrocytes.

Most antibody forming cells probably live for only a few days. A small proportion last for weeks or months.

Antibody production in the spleen after an intravenous injection of antigen follows a similar pattern. It is interesting that a small number of antibody–plaque forming cells of many specificities can be found in spleens from apparently unimmunized mice, probably because of chronic stimulation by cross-reacting antigens from the environment. Repeated injection of an antigen also induces some antibody formation in bone marrow and lungs.

As well as class changes during the course of an immune response, there is usually a gradual and substantial increase in the average affinity for antigen of the serum antibody. Reasons for this are discussed in Section 6.6.

4.8 ANTIBODY FEEDBACK

Why does antibody production stop? If it did not, the animal would obviously become full of specific antibody. One mechanism is a simple feedback loop: the removal of the stimulating antigen by antibody (the end product). (IgG is particularly efficient while IgM antibody may actually enhance responses, for reasons which are not clear.) However, there is much more to the regulation of immune responses than this, as we shall see in Chapter 11.

4.9 CLONAL PROLIFERATION OF ANTIBODY FORMING CELLS

After appropriate stimulation with antigen (Chapter 5) a B lymphocyte proliferates and differentiates to generate a *clone* of antibody forming cells. [A clone (Section 3.1) means all the descendants of one cell produced by mitotic division.] It first transforms, without dividing, into a large blast cell, which then, on division, typically gives rise to smaller more basophilic mononuclear cells, and finally to plasma cells (Fig. 4.14). Other developmental sequences also exist: the situation is very complex. Estimates of the average time between cell divisions vary, but are mostly around 12 hours.

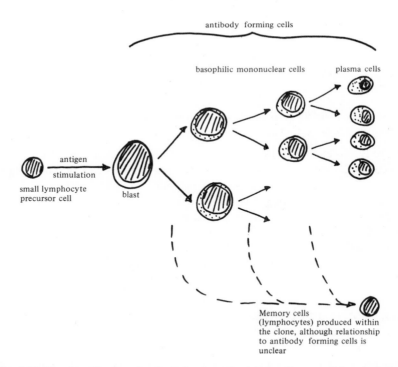

Fig. 4.14 Clonal proliferation of antibody forming cells. A "clone" means all the mitotic descendants of a single cell. Individual clones from one B lymphocyte may eventually have some thousands of members.

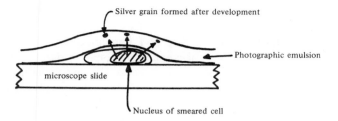

Fig. 4.15 Autoradiography. The DNA of the smeared cell has previously taken up a radioactive label, e.g., in tritiated thymidine. β emissions strike the photographic emulsion above the cell, and silver grains may be developed in these areas of the emulsion.

Evidence for this life history comes from experiments where a DNA label, usually tritiated thymidine, is injected into an antigenically stimulated animal. Antibody forming cells are identified, e.g., by micromanipulative or fluorescent antibody techniques, then these cells are examined for the presence of DNA label by autoradiography (Fig. 4.15). This tells whether or not the antibody forming cell has synthesized new DNA since the tritiated thymidine was administered. Comparison of labeled cells immediately and several hours after injection of label shows that the cells labeled only at the later time period must have arisen by division from the early labeled population. Thus a developmental sequence can be pieced together.

Methods have been devised for identifying single clones of antibody forming cells. It is currently impossible to say how many divisions a single clone undergoes during a normal response, since all methods for studying them involve their isolation in some way from other clones, e.g., in tissue culture (Section 5.4.1), and the growth of a clone is certainly strongly influenced by the density and behavior of neighboring cells. However, it is clear that clones may potentially vary in size from very few to as many as 50,000 or more cells. Clones begin by producing IgM antibody, but, as mentioned above, there is probably a switch at some stage to production of IgG antibody with the same specificity (some debate still surrounds this question of Ig class switch).

4.10 SUMMARY

Small lymphocytes are metabolically quiescent cells, many of which recirculate continuously around the body, passing out of the blood into the lymphatic circulation within lymph nodes and other organized lymphoid tissue in spleen and gut wall. There are two broad categories of lymphocyte: T cells, which come from the thymus, and B cells, from the bone marrow (in adult mammals). Foreign antigens localize in lymphoid tissue and there stimulate a proportion of lymphocytes to proliferate and differentiate into "effector" cells, antibody forming cells in the case of the B line of lymphocytes, and a variety of antigen-sensitive and regulatory cells in the case of T lymphocytes.

Antibody forming cells appear in stimulated lymphoid tissue within a few days. They can be identified by a variety of techniques, including immunofluorescence, micromanipulative procedures, and the hemolytic plaque technique. Most antibody formers are plasma cells or basophilic lymphoid mononuclear cells of various sizes. Each produces antibody of a single specificity and (usually at least) of only one Ig class. A single B lymphocyte, on appropriate stimulation with antigen, proliferates and differentiates to form a clone of antibody forming cells which may have several thousand members.

FURTHER READING

4.1   Bessis, M. (1973). "Living Blood Cells and Their Ultrastructure." (Translated by R. I. Weed.) Springer-Verlag, Berlin, Heidelberg, New York.
4.2   Cunningham, A. J. (1973). Antibody formation studied at the single cell level. *Prog. Allergy* **17**, 5. Reviews techniques, and evidence that cells make only one kind of antibody.
4.3   Cunningham, A. J. (1977). Gestalt Immunology: a less reductionist approach to the subject. *In* "Theoretical Immunology" (G. Bell, A. Perelson, and G. Pimbley, eds.), in press. Marcel Dekker, New York.
4.4   Ford, W. L. (1975). Lymphocyte migration and immune responses. *Prog. Allergy* **19**, 1.
4.5   Greaves, M. F., Owen, J., and Raff, M. (1973). "T and B Lymphocytes: Their Origins, Properties and Roles in Immune Responses." North Holland, Amsterdam.
4.6   McGregor, D. D. and Gowans, J. L. (1963). The antibody response of rats depleted of lymphocytes by chronic drainage from the thoracic duct. *J. Exp. Med.* **117**, 303.
4.7   Metcalf, D. and Moore, M. A. S. (1971). "Haemopoietic Cells." North Holland, Amsterdam.
4.8   Nossal, G. J. V. and Ada, G. L. (1971). "Antigens, Lymphoid Cells, and the Immune Response." Academic Press, New York. Contains details on the localization of antigens in lymphoid tissue.
4.9   Nossal G. J. V. and Makela, O. (1962). Elaboration of antibody by single cells. *Annu. Rev. Microbiol.* **16**, 53. Reviews the classic early work on this subject.

QUESTIONS

4.1   Sheep and goat red blood cells (RBC) show extensive serological cross-reactivity (about 25%) in mice, i.e., if a mouse is immunized against sheep RBC, the serum hemolytic titer against goat RBC will be about one-quarter of that against sheep. Suppose such an immunized mouse had 10^5 anti-sheep RBC antibody plaque forming cells in its spleen (Section 4.5.2). What would you expect to find if a plaque test was done on (a) goat RBC; (b) on a mixed indicator layer of sheep plus goat RBC?

4.2   How might you test the idea that an immune response stops because of the production of antibody which then removes the antigenic stimulus? How would the inhibitory capacity of the various classes of antibody be tested?

4.3   It is possible to cannulate (insert a fine plastic tube into) the efferent lymphatic vessel issuing from the popliteal lymph node of a sheep. The cells coming out of the node can then be collected and examined over a period of weeks. Normal rate of flow is about $2 - 5 \times 10^6$ cells per hour, and these cells are mainly small- or medium-sized lymphocytes. After injecting antigen subcutaneously into an area of the lower leg from which lymph drains into the popliteal node, the output of cells in its efferent lymph increases about tenfold. What new kinds of cell would you expect to find in the efferent lymph after such antigenic stimulation of the node? Where do these extra cells come from and how would you demonstrate this?

Immunocompetent Cells and Induction of the Antibody Response

5.1 IMMUNOCOMPETENT CELLS

A glance back to Fig. 4.7 reminds us of the important distinction between "effector" cells of the T or B lines, and "precursor" cells, those able to be activated by antigen to produce more differentiated progeny. The term *immunocompetent cell* strictly refers to those T or B lymphocytes which, while not yet making an active immune response, are capable of being immediately stimulated by antigen to generate effector offspring. "Precursor" is really a more general word: the hemopoietic stem cell (Section 4.2.2) is a precursor of lymphocytes; the zygote is a precursor of all cells in the body. The initials "T" and "B" are used fairly loosely, sometimes to refer only to immunocompetent precursor lymphocytes, and sometimes to indicate all members of a cell lineage.

In the previous chapter we have briefly discussed the events between the stimulation by antigen of an immunocompetent B cell and its proliferation to the antibody forming cell stage. We will now move back a step and look at the properties of this B cell. We will then examine how such cells are induced to start differentiating, a complex and interesting process which involves *cooperation* between T lymphocytes, B lymphocytes, and macrophages.

5.2 THE IMMUNOCOMPETENT B CELL

Two related properties of these cells are particularly important:

(a) They are *committed* or *restricted,* before meeting antigen, to make only one kind of antibody.

(b) They react with antigen through specific, cell surface-bound immuno-globulin receptor molecules which have the same specificity as the antibody their immediate descendants will secrete, a "sample of their wares" as it were.

5.2.1 Evidence for Ig Receptors

Anti-Ig antibodies have various effects when allowed to interact with the surface of immunocompetent B cells. When intact cells are treated with fluorescein-labeled anti-Ig, those with surface Ig can be distinguished (Section 4.5.1). Some B lymphocytes can be induced to transform into blasts by anti-Ig, which appears to act like an antigen on their surface receptor molecules (see also Section 5.2.4). Anti-immunoglobulin antibody plus complement may lyse receptor bearing B lymphocytes and, in so doing, destroy the subsequent ability of the population to make antibody. The surface immunoglobulins of immunocompetent cells have also been labeled (e.g., biosynthetically, by "feeding" cells with radioisotope-labeled amino acids), and then isolated and characterized following solubilization of the plasma membrane in various ways.

5.2.2 Evidence for Specific Antigen Binding by Surface Ig Receptors

If a population of lymphoid cells is treated with a specific antigen, a small proportion of them will bind it to their surfaces, as can be conveniently demonstrated if the antigen is labeled in some way. Radioisotope-labeled soluble antigen has commonly been used in this kind of work, antigen-binding cells then being detected by autoradiography (Section 4.9). Fluorescence staining can also be employed. In a similar way, a small proportion of immunocompetent lymphocytes will bind foreign erythrocytes forming "rosettes," clusters of the erythrocytes around a central lymphocyte. It is standard practice in this kind of work to demonstrate that binding of antigen can be inhibited by pretreating the cells with anti-Ig, thus reassuring the experimenter that attachment of antigen took place through an Ig receptor molecule.

The number of cells detected as binding a specific antigen is much smaller than the number with surface Ig, which implies diversity among cells in their antigen binding specificities. Approximately one-half of the cells in mouse spleen have surface Ig. Typically one cell in ten thousand might bind a soluble protein antigen presented at low concentration. Interestingly, as the concentration of antigen applied to the cells is raised, the number of binding cells increases, up to 1–2% at high antigen concentrations (several micrograms per milliliter). This reflects a range in the *affinities* of the cell receptors for antigen: at low concentrations only those with high affinity will trap the antigen; at higher concentrations, some antigen is attached even to receptors which bind it weakly.

The binding of antigen by cells can be exploited to remove lymphocytes with particular specificities from a population of cells. For example, cells may be filtered through a column containing antigen attached to a solid support in a method analogous to the affinity chromatography of molecules, when cells of that particular antigen reactivity will be removed from the population, while the ability to react against unrelated antigens is not affected (Fig. 5.1).

The binding of radioactive antigen to cells can also be used to rid a population selectively of specific precursor cells [the "suicide" technique of Ada (Fig. 5.2)]. Highly radioactive antigen (X) is mixed with lymphoid cells and left at 0°C for several hours. The antigen attaches only to those cells with anti-X receptors. These are now killed by the localized irradiation; an isotope such as ^{125}I, whose emissions have a short path length, is used to restrict the effect to the cells actually binding antigen. When this cell suspension is washed and tested for its ability to react to X and a control antigen, C, it responds only to C (Fig. 5.2; Table 5.1). As a further refinement, cells may be exposed to anti-Ig serum before adding the radioactive antigen; under some circumstances this will protect the cells from suicide, again showing that the receptor molecules were probably Ig in nature (Ref. 5.1).

5.2.3 Number and Class of Receptor Molecules

Estimates of the number of Ig molecules on a B cell vary widely: there are of the order of 10^5 identical receptors per cell. They are slowly shed from the

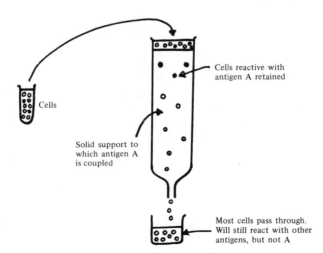

Fig. 5.1 Affinity chromatography of lymphoid cells.

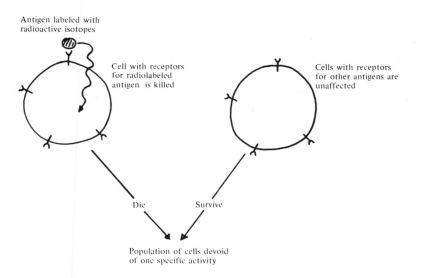

Fig. 5.2 "Suicide" of cells binding radioactive antigen.

plasma membrane and resynthesized, at a rate estimated as around 20 molecules per minute per cell.

The class of receptor Ig is currently the subject of some debate. It is clear that IgM receptors occur on many B lymphocytes; the molecule is not, however, in the polymeric 19 S form (Section 3.2), but exists in the membrane as a 7-8 S

TABLE 5.1

Antibody Titers Made by Mouse Spleen Cells after Pretreatment with Radioactive or Nonradioactive Antigens[a]

Antigenic pretreatment	Radioactivity of pretreatment antigen	Mean antibody titer ($\log_2$) after challenge with	
		X	Y
X	+	0.5	5.4
X	−	2.9	4.3
Y	+	2.0	1.1
Y	−	3.3	4.2
No antigen		2.3	4.7

[a]X and Y were non-cross-reacting bacterial antigens. Cells were injected into groups of irradiated recipient mice (Section 5.4.1), then challenged with either the antigen used in the pretreatment step, or with the other antigen. Depressive effects were only seen when the pretreatment antigen was radioactive, and the same as the challenge antigen. (Data from Ada and Byrt, Ref. 5.1.)

monomer lacking the terminal galactose, fucose, and N-acetylneuraminic acid carbohydrate residues of the normal μ chains. Recently a new class of Ig, IgD (Section 3.2) which is rare in the serum, has been recognized on the surface of a large proportion of mature B lymphocytes. IgM and IgD often occur together on the same cell.

There is some evidence that memory B cells, that is lymphocytes generated after antigenic stimulation (Chapter 6), bear IgG or IgA receptors. It was thought that the receptor mimicked the eventual product of the cell both in specificity and class: that a cell destined to generate IgG antibody forming progeny, for example, would have IgG receptors. This has not been disproved, but it seems that some earlier identifications of receptors as IgG or IgA may have been incorrect, for two reasons: (1) sera used to characterize these receptors, and supposedly anti-γ or anti-α chain in specificity, may have been cross-reacting with the δ chains of IgD; (2) B cells have a receptor for the Fc part of IgG, as do macrophages (Section 4.2.4). It may have been such superficially bound IgG which was diagnosed as receptor material. It is possible that most or all true receptor molecules on B cells will turn out to be IgM or IgD; why the two kinds should be needed is not yet clear (Ref. 5.19).

5.2.4 The Reaction of Cell Surface Receptors with Antigen

Like other cell surface proteins, the Ig receptor molecules are "floating" in the phospholipid bilayer which constitutes the plasma membrane. Receptors can thus be clumped together by polyvalent antigens or anti-Ig, and these clumps appear as "patches" if the antigen is labeled, for example, with a fluorescent dye. At 37°C these patches "cap," i.e., coalesce and move to one pole of the cell where the antigen–receptor complexes are endocytosed (taken into the cytoplasm). This dramatic event must have biological significance, but exactly what is currently unknown. B cells from adult mice resynthesize their receptors 5–20 hours after capping, whereas those from fetal or neonatal mice do not, a finding which some have interpreted to mean that B cells from young animals are inactivated ("tolerized," Chapter 6) rather than stimulated by an antigen with which they come in contact.

Appropriate interaction with antigen is the *specific* event which triggers a cell. It seems likely that cross-linking ("patching"?) of receptors is somehow important in "signaling" this contact to the cytoplasm. Events within the cytoplasm, i.e., the further passage of messages to the DNA that provoke transcription are still unclear, but are likely to be the same as in other cell types induced by hormones or other microenvironmental stimuli.

5.2.5 Development of B Lymphocytes

In the last chapter we encountered the bursa of Fabricius, a small primary lymphoid organ in birds, derived, like the thymus, from gut epithelium and situated adjacent to the cloaca (Section 4.2.2). This organ seems to be entirely responsible for inducing more primitive lymphoid cells, which lodge in it, to differentiate into Ig-bearing B lymphocytes. Removal of the bursa (bursectomy) within a few days after hatching drastically impairs the bird's subsequent ability to make Ig and specific antibody, without affecting thymus functions (Chapter 9). The bursa continues to provide B lymphocytes into adult life, involuting only after sexual maturity.

In mammals there is no organ known to be exactly equivalent to the bursa. The fetal liver may, however, have the same function for at least some time in the development of mammals; in mice, which have been most studied, it is a large hemopoietic organ that is seeded by Ig negative cells and generates Ig-positive lymphocytes, the first of these, according to recent reports, appearing at about day 13 of the 20-day gestation period. B lymphocytes with larger amounts of surface Ig are first detected around day 17, and occur simultaneously in liver, spleen, and bone marrow. In mice, after birth, the liver loses all hemopoietic function, which is now assumed by bone marrow (discussed further in Ref. 4.7).

The bone marrow of an adult mouse turns out approximately 10^8 Ig-bearing small B lymphocytes per day. It is not clear whether parts of the bone marrow are acting like the bursa and (probably) the fetal liver, i.e., as primary inductive lymphoid tissue, or whether the bone marrow is simply a factory for multiplying lymphocytes which have already received their critical inductive stimulus from the liver in fetal life. This interesting question is lent added piquancy by recent experiments in which destruction of most of the bone marrow (by local irradiation from radioactive strontium, taken up selectively by bone) made little difference to the B lymphocyte supply in mice; evidently they can be produced at other sites as well, particularly in the spleen.

The first B lymphocytes in developing mice have IgM receptors only; cells bearing both M and D do not appear until about 10 days after birth. The baby mouse responds very poorly to injected antigens until around this time, but it would probably by unwise to draw the obvious correlation between function and receptor structure since much of the unresponsiveness of newborn rodents has recently been shown to be caused by overwhelming production of suppressor T lymphocytes (Chapter 11) in these young animals.

Figure 5.3 is a tentative scheme for the development of B cells. Lymphocytes can be fractionated by size according to the rate at which they sediment through a liquid medium when allowed to stand for some hours (Ref. 5.10); similarly they can be divided into different density categories by centrifugation to equilibrium in a density gradient (Fig. 5.4). For example, evidence for the small size of mature B lymphocytes (Fig. 5.3), comes from experiments in which cells were separated by size, the different fractions being then tested for ability to generate antibody forming cells on appropriate culture (Section 5.4.1). Generally speaking, dividing, differentiating cells tend to be larger and less dense, while lymphocytes which are not engaged in any active immunological function (but are

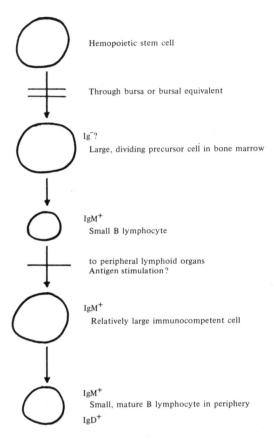

Hemopoietic stem cell

Through bursa or bursal equivalent

Ig^-?
Large, dividing precursor cell in bone marrow

IgM^+
Small B lymphocyte

to peripheral lymphoid organs
Antigen stimulation?

IgM^+
Relatively large immunocompetent cell

IgM^+
Small, mature B lymphocyte in periphery
IgD^+

Fig. 5.3 Tentative developmental sequence for mammalian B lymphocytes.

instead ''waiting'' to be activated by antigen) tend to be smaller and more dense. Small Ig-bearing B cells come from larger dividing precursors in bone marrow. There is recent evidence, still controversial, that these small lymphocytes, whatever their specificity, may commonly be stimulated by cross-reacting environmental antigens on reaching peripheral lymphoid tissue, with the result that the population of immunocompetent B cells in lymph nodes and spleen consists of a mixture of cells of varying sizes and degrees of activity. The full development of peripheral lymphoid tissue, and of normal levels of serum Ig, seems to depend on the kind of chronic and constant antigenic bombardment which most animals experience. By contrast, the *lymphopoietic* (lymphocyte producing) activity of primary lymphoid organs is independent of environmental antigen.

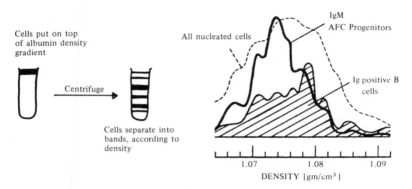

Fig. 5.4 Separation of mouse spleen cells according to density, by centrifugation in a gradient of isosmotic albumin. After all cells had reached equilibrium (i.e., had arrived at that part of the gradient where the albumin was as dense as themselves), sequential fractions were collected from the tube. Each fraction was then tested in three ways: for the total number of cells it contained; for the number of Ig$^+$ cells; and for the relative number of cells capable of giving an IgM antibody response when stimulated with antigen in an irradiated recipient mouse (Section 5.4.1). The three curves represent the distribution of these three activities down the gradient (from Fidler, Howard, and Shortman, Ref. 5.6).

5.3 THE IMMUNOCOMPETENT T CELL

The properties of T cells are less precisely known than those of the B line, a deficiency which seems likely to be soon remedied by the vigorous and widespread research effort currently being devoted to them. T cells deserve a chapter to themselves (Chapter 9), but to clear the way for further discussion on induction of B cells we need to summarize the main properties of their cooperating T partners:

1. T cells have developmental history analogous to that of B cells; they are derived from uncommitted stem cells which migrate into the thymus, and proliferate and differentiate there, yielding large numbers of T lymphocytes. Some of these escape into the recirculating pool and peripheral lymphoid organs.

2. Like B cells, T cells are diverse in their specificity, and are thought to be committed to the synthesis of only one kind of receptor before meeting antigen.

3. The nature of T cell receptors is currently under intense study; they are probably Ig or Ig-like molecules but much less numerous than on B cells. (Chapter 9).

4. T cells have a variety of functions, some of which have nothing to do with B cells. They also play an important role in regulating the induction of B cells, and we are for the moment concerned with these "helper" properties (below).

5. T cells have a characteristic antigen called θ (recently renamed "Thy-1") on their surface, against which antiserum may be raised. Such anti-θ serum can be used to kill selectively all the T cells in a population. Anti-θ serum is usually made by immunizing one strain of mice repeatedly with thymus cells from another strain which has a slightly different antigenic type of θ.

5.4 CELL COOPERATION IN THE INDUCTION OF ANTIBODY FORMATION

One of the most exciting events in modern immunology has been the way in which two quite separate lines of research have led to the same important conclusion, that collaboration between specific T and B cells is needed for induction of antibody formation. The two kinds of experiment are work with mixtures of thymus and bone marrow cells, and studies on the immune response to simple haptens. We will look at both of these, but first it is necessary to discuss methods of studying the immune response of *defined* cell populations.

5.4.1 Culturing Lymphoid Cells

Measuring the serum antibody response of an animal to injected antigen can provide a lot of information about the activities of lymphoid cells, but it is not possible to control the number or kinds of cells stimulated by the antigen. For example, the relative numbers of T and B cells involved can not be manipulated experimentally. This lack of flexibility is common to "whole animal" work in many subjects. To answer some questions, a more analytical approach is needed.

5.4.1.1 *In Vitro cultures of antibody forming cells*

Obviously if it were possible to take a known number of lymphoid cells and induce them to produce antibody in a test tube, then we would have an experimental system which was more suited to manipulation than is the whole animal. Cell culture with some cell types (e.g., fibroblasts) has been practiced since the beginning of this century. Growing highly differentiated cells is much more difficult, and primary antigenic stimulation of antibody forming cell production from B cells was not achieved *in vitro* until a few years ago (Mishell and Dutton, Ref. 5.11). The basic technique consists of incubating lymphoid cells at high density in a petri dish which is slowly and continuously rocked. The medium contains fetal calf serum, and is in equilibrium with a gas mixture of 7% O_2, 10% CO_2, and N_2.

Variants of this technique exist. A particularly useful method involves dividing the cell suspension into a number of microcultures (Lefkovits, Ref. 5.7, and Marbrook and Haskill, Ref. 5.8). Figure 5.5 shows a culture vessel which has 36

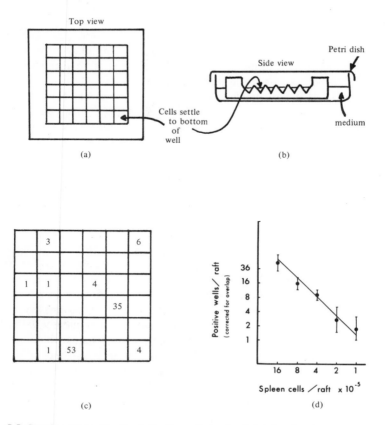

Fig. 5.5 Growing clones of antibody forming cells *in vitro* in Marbrook polyacrylamide "rafts." (a) and (b) show top and side views of a raft, which has 36 wells. Cells settle into the wells, and each becomes an independent microculture. (c) After culturing a total of 4 × 10⁵ cells for 3 days, these were the numbers of anti-sheep erythrocyte antibody forming cells in each well: blanks mean no plaque forming cells (unpublished data from L. M. Pilarski and A. J. Cunningham). (d) The number of wells containing one or more antibody forming cells after culturing varying numbers of mouse spleen cells for 2 days (from Pilarski and Cunningham Ref. 5.15).

individual wells. Approximately 10^4–10^5 normal mouse spleen cells are allowed to settle into each well, and the culture is incubated for 2 to 4 days at 37°C with sheep erythrocytes as antigen. After this culture period, each microculture is separately assayed for hemolytic plaque forming cells. Some wells have up to about 100 antibody forming cells, while others have none.

A lot of information can be gathered from such experiments. Under suitable conditions, we can infer that each "positive" well contains a clone of mitotic descendants from a single, precursor B cell. The size these clones reach in a given time, and the rate of division, are readily calculated. The frequency of B cells able to respond to a particular antigen can be estimated, e.g., if there were 10^4 cells per well, and only one well in ten produced any plaque forming cells, the frequency of B cells in the population able to respond to sheep erythrocyte antigen would be 1 in 10^5. The number of specific B cells detected by such *functional* tests is always much lower than the number which *bind* the same antigen (Section 5.2.2). One reason for this discrepancy is that cells with quite low affinity receptors can make firm multivalent attachments to antigen, as we have seen, without subsequently producing individual antibody molecules of high enough affinity to have a detectable effect on the antigen (in this case, erythrocyte lysis). These clonal cultures can also be used to compare the frequency of precursor cells in unprimed animals (often quaintly called "virgin" B cells) and in primed animals, where they are usually at least ten times more numerous.

5.4.1.2 *Adoptive transfer*

A second method for "culturing" populations of lymphocytes has been in general use for longer (~15 years) than the *in vitro* techniques. A mouse (or other animal) is given a sufficiently high dose of γ- or X-irradiation (about 800 r) to destroy its ability to respond to antigen. (Irradiation exerts this effect by so severely damaging chromosomes that any cell which subsequently divides will die.) Lymphoid cells from a normal animal are now injected, with antigen, into this irradiated "host," which regains some immune responsiveness "by adoption" (Fig. 5.6). It is usual either to measure the serum antibody produced by such animals or to count numbers of plaque forming cells appearing in their spleens. The irradiated host acts as a sort of test tube which provides favorable conditions for the growth of the injected cells. These cells must come from the same inbred strain of animals as their new host otherwise a graft versus host reaction may occur (Section 10.6).

5.4.2 Thymus/Bone Marrow Cell Cooperation

The first evidence that the thymus plays an important part in antibody formation came in 1962 (Ref. 5.9) when Miller showed that removing the thymus from a newborn mouse (neonatal thymectomy) greatly depressed its ability to respond

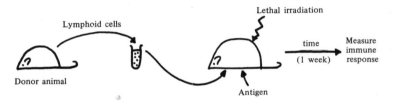

Fig. 5.6 Adoptive transfer technique.

to many antigens during the rest of its life. This agreed well with observations in human clinical medicine: babies born without a thymus or with various thymic deficiencies are poor antibody producers.

The next important advance was made in 1966 when Claman and his collaborators (Ref. 5.3) found that irradiated mice injected with a mixture of thymus and bone marrow cells could produce far more antibody to sheep erythrocyte antigen than control groups of mice given only one of the two lymphoid cell types. Davies, and Miller and his associates showed that it was the cell from bone marrow in such mixtures which produced the antibody: the thymus cell was acting as a "helper." This important result came from experiments where marked cells were used; e.g., the mice donating thymus and bone marrow cells were of different types. Antisera could be produced which destroyed one type and not the other (Fig. 5.7).

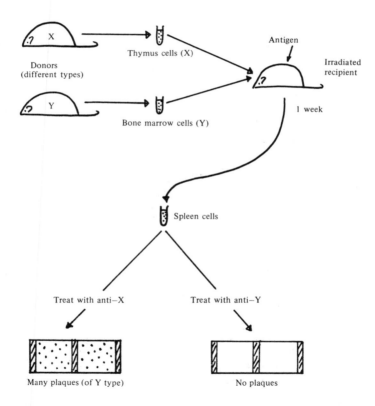

Fig. 5.7 Cell collaboration: identifying the source of antibody forming cells. Donors X and Y have lymphocytes with different surface antigens against which specific antisera can be made. All plaque forming cells from the thymus/bone marrow mixture carried the antigens characteristic of the mouse donating the bone marrow.

How the thymus cells helped the response was not clear from these experiments. One possibility was that the presence of thymus cells simply provided more favorable conditions in a nonspecific way for the cells from bone marrow to differentiate. This was ruled out by the elegant thymus cell "education" (activation) experiment of Miller, which demonstrated that those thymus cells involved in cooperation react *specifically* with the antigen. Miller essentially split Claman's experiment into two parts (Fig. 5.8). The thymus cells were first injected

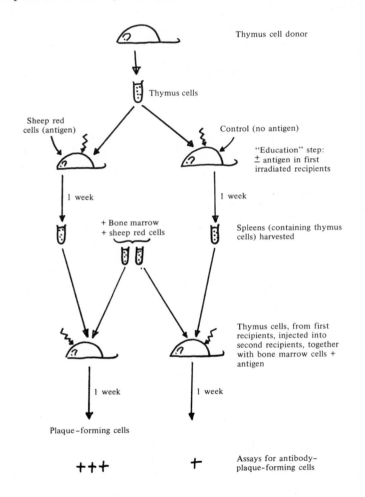

Fig. 5.8 Thymus cell "education" experiment; more antibody forming cells were produced by mice receiving bone marrow together with thymus cells which had already been in contact with the specific antigen.

alone into irradiated hosts. These mice received either the test antigen (sheep red blood cells) or a control, non-cross-reacting antigen (horse red blood cells). After 1 week, the spleens were collected, and used as a source of thymus-derived cells for injection into a second host, this time mixed with bone marrow. It was found that the initial "education" period in the first host substantially increased the overall response of the second mouse, provided the sheep erythrocyte antigen was used in both cases. The current interpretation of this experiment is that antigen stimulates clonal proliferation of committed T cells in the first host, so that much larger numbers of helper T cells specific for the antigen are transferred to the second host and are then better able to stimulate specific bone marrow B cells.

5.4.3 The Hapten–Carrier System

It will be recalled (from Section 2.3.2) that a hapten is a small molecular weight compound which will not induce an immune response when injected by itself, but will, if coupled to a carrier protein, induce antibody molecules which react specifically with the hapten. The hapten acts as an extra determinant (Section 2.3.1) on the molecule, and the response to the hapten can be experimentally distinguished from the response to the rest of the molecule. The amount of antibody made during a primary response to a hapten–protein conjugate is usually small, but after a secondary injection of the same compound, much more antibody is produced: this is because of clonal proliferation by B cells able to react with the antigen (and see next chapter on "memory").

It was found (Benacerraf) that in order to get a good secondary response to a hapten, it had to be reinjected coupled to the *same* protein as for the primary response. This interesting finding focused attention on the possible role played by the rest of the molecule in assisting a response to the haptenic portion. An early proposal was the *local environment* hypothesis (Fig. 5.9) which held that a cell stimulated by a hapten had to "recognize" not only the haptenic group, but also some of the surrounding protein. Mitchison (Ref. 5.13) showed that this was not a complete explanation, and at the same time demonstrated the need for two different cells to react with an antigen in order to induce an immune response to it. Figure 5.10 shows one of his experiments. One mouse was immunized with hapten–protein X, the other with protein Y alone. Cells from both animals were mixed and injected into an irradiated recipient. Stimulating this recipient with hapten–protein Y now gave as much anti-hapten antibody as hapten–protein X would have done (Table 5.2 and Fig. 5.10). It has since been confirmed that the carrier-primed helper cells (i.e., those from the animal injected with protein Y in Fig. 5.10) in such experiments are sensitive to anti-θ serum and therefore are T cells, while the hapten-primed precursor cells (exposed to hapten–protein X) are not sensitive to anti-θ serum and belong to the B line (Table 5.3). What appears

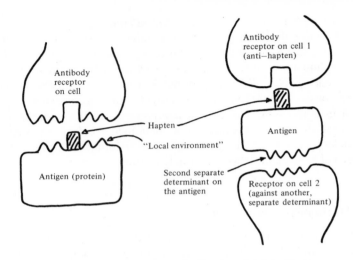

Fig. 5.9 Local environment and cell cooperation hypotheses.

to be happening is that T cells primed against the protein are helping the response of B cells with specificity for the hapten, a demonstration of synergism which has obvious similarities to the thymus/bone marrow work.

The hapten and the "new" carrier ("Y" in these experiments) must be coupled together: injection of the irradiated recipient animal (Fig. 5.6) with hapten–protein Z together with protein Y will not usually induce much anti-hapten antibody (Table 5.2). It seems that the helper T cell must produce something which can interact with the antigen molecules whose haptenic residues are already bound to the B cell (see next section).

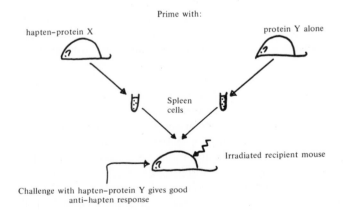

Fig. 5.10 Hapten-carrier protein cell cooperation.

TABLE 5.2
Typical Hapten-Carrier Experiment

	Cells induced	
Priming antigens	T	B
Mouse (1) Hap-protein X	Anti-hap, Anti-X	Anti-hap, Anti-X
Mouse (2) Protein Y	Anti-Y	Anti-Y

Effect of different kinds of antigen challenge[a]

Antigen challenge	Cells involved in making anti-hapten antibody	Size of anti-hapten response
Hap-protein X	T cells anti-X B cells anti-hap	+++
Hap-protein Y	T cells anti-Y B cells anti-hap	+++
Hap-protein Z	No T cells B cells anti-hap	−

[a] After cells from (1) and (2) are mixed.

TABLE 5.3
Cooperation between Hapten-Primed B Cells and Carrier-Primed T Cells[a]

Group[b]	Description of the treatment	B cells NIP-CGG primed	Pretreatment of B cells	T cells	Pretreatment of T cells	Antigen challenge NIP-BSA	Anti-NIP response
1	T + B, no Ag	+	None	+	None	None	1.2
2	T + B + Ag	+	None	+	None	+	100.0
3	T only, + Ag	None	None	+	None	+	1.7
4	B only, + Ag	+	None	None	None	+	18.6
5	B + T (anti-θ treated) + Ag	+	None	+	Anti-θ	+	5.4
6	T + B (anti-θ treated) + Ag	+	Anti-θ	+	None	+	97.7

[a] Primed B cells were obtained from mice immunized with 4-hydroxy-3-iodo-5-nitrophenylacetic acid (NIP, a hapten) coupled to chicken γ-globulin (CGG), giving "NIP-CGG." Primed T cells came from mice immunized with bovine serum albumin, BSA. The cells were mixed and injected into irradiated recipient mice together with a challenge antigen consisting of NIP-BSA, the hapten coupled to the "new" carrier (see text). The anti-NIP response of these recipient mice is expressed as moles of NIP bound per milliliter of serum ($\times 10^{-9}$).

[b] Comparison of groups 1 and 2 shows the 100-fold effect of antigenic challenge. Groups 3 and 4 received only "primed T" or "primed B" cells (both would have contained unprimed T and B cells, which accounts for their small, positive responses). Comparing groups 2 and 5 shows the depressive effect of pretreating the carrier-primed cells with anti-θ serum, while the lack of effect of this serum on hapten-primed cells can be seen in group 6. (Data calculated from Raff, Ref. 5.16.)

It is worth emphasizing that both T and B cells are stimulated by a protein injected alone, but the use of haptenic determinants that can be coupled to different proteins allows the experimental separation of two separate populations of cells reacting to different parts of the same complex molecule. Similarly, the hapten and the protein each probably stimulate both B and T cells, but in these experiments it is the helper function of anti-protein cells and antibody function of anti-hapten cells to which attention is directed.

5.5 MECHANISMS OF CELL COOPERATION

The means by which specific T cells help B cells to differentiate for antibody formation is now seen as part of a larger question: How do certain T cells regulate, in both enhancing and inhibitory ways, the immune reactions of B and other T cells? Detailed mechanisms are still uncertain, and probably complex. This area of research is currently in a state of turmoil. Many different "factors" have been isolated from lymphocytes and shown to have various effects on other lymphocytes, but it is extremely difficult to know how these are related to *in vivo* mechanisms operating during a normal immune response. We will review this question Chapter 11, and for the present will confine ourselves to outlining the main principles likely to operate in these cell interactions.

5.5.1 Role of the Macrophage

The players in this drama include not only T and B lymphocytes, but also macrophages. Tissue culture studies show that removing macrophages (by allowing them to stick to glass then separating the nonadherent lymphocytes) often drastically decreases immune responses. Clumps of lymphocytes around a central macrophage have been observed microscopically in samples taken from tissue cultures engaged in immune responses; breaking up such clumps early in a response may diminish it. Cytoplasmic channels between macrophages and lymphocytes can sometimes be seen in fixed preparations from lymphoid tissue. *In vivo,* as we discussed in Section 4.3, complex changes in organization (e.g., follicle formation) and traffic of lymphocytes in peripheral lymphoid organs accompany any immune response. Macrophages appear not only to break up large antigenic particles, but also to "present" antigen in small amounts on their outer surfaces. One of the frustrating aspects of work on cell interactions is that it is virtually impossible to duplicate normal lymphoid tissue organization in tissue culture systems, yet is is equally difficult to understand detailed mechanisms without using simple, experimental models.

5.5.2 Formation of an Antigen Matrix

There seem to be two broad kinds of mechanisms which are likely to be important in lymphocyte–lymphocyte–macrophage interactions. The first of these is *matrix* formation, that is, the polymerizing of small antigen molecules into larger units on the surface of a B cell, which has the effect of "patching" the lymphocyte's receptors in localized areas (Section 5.2.4). There is some evidence that appropriate receptor aggregation is by itself sufficient to trigger proliferation and differentiation in a B cell. In any case, we have seen (Section 2.3.3) how such multivalent combinations produce exponential increases in the strength of binding between antigen and cell. A very small antigen can not induce a cell because there is no way it can cross-link receptors or draw two cells together [Fig. 5.11 part (a)]. A larger molecule which is asymmetric, and possesses only one determinant of any one kind, also cannot cross-link receptors [part (b)]. Such molecules (bovine serum albumin is an example), are very *thymus dependent*. They induce antibody responses only in the presence of large numbers of specifically activated T cells. Molecules which are highly polymeric with respect to a single determinant, such as pneumococcal polysaccharide, polyvinylpyrrolidone, or D-amino acid polymers, are much less thymus dependent (some would say completely *independent* although it is difficult to establish that T cells are ever totally lacking in a population of lymphocytes). Figure 5.11 part (c) shows how these molecules can bind strongly by multivalent combination. However, as we can see from part (d) of this figure, antigens with several different determinants can be linked together in a matrix by antibody directed at "carrier" segments of the molecule. This kind of array might be most efficiently built up on the surface of another cell. There is some evidence that T cells release antibody-like factors which bind to macrophages and "present" antigen to B cells in this way.

5.5.3 A Second Signal

The other major kind of mechanism currently postulated is the delivery of a *second signal* from a helper T cell or macrophage to the B lymphocyte that is to be induced [Fig. 5.11 part (a)], a "first" signal having been provided by bound antigen. The transmission of such a signal might depend on drawing two immunocompetent cells together around an antigen "sandwich." Alternatively, the final helper cell might be a macrophage which had first bound, on its surface, antibody or an antibody-like material made by the T cell. Another possibility is that the second signal might be provided by the "Fc" equivalent part of the antigen binding molecules secreted by the T cell [Fig. 5.11 part (f)]. Note that while any such second signal is likely to be nonspecific, that is, the same whatever the antigen, the initial stimulation of both T and B cells depends on their binding specifically to the particular antigen used to elicit the response.

Both of these effects may be involved in B cell induction, and similar mechanisms are now thought to be needed for inducing effector T cells as well (Chapter 9). It is interesting that production of different classes of antibody requires a different amount of T cell help. IgM antibody against many antigens can be made in the presence of minimal numbers of T cells. IgG and IgE need more T cells. An obviously related fact is that polymeric antigens tend to be

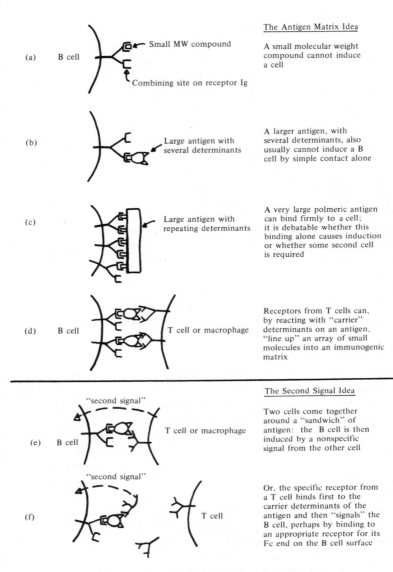

The Antigen Matrix Idea

(a) B cell — Small MW compound — Combining site on receptor Ig

A small molecular weight compound cannot induce a cell

(b) Large antigen with several determinants

A larger antigen, with several determinants, also usually cannot induce a B cell by simple contact alone

(c) Large antigen with repeating determinants

A very large polmeric antigen can bind firmly to a cell; it is debatable whether this binding alone causes induction or whether some second cell is required

(d) B cell — T cell or macrophage

Receptors from T cells can, by reacting with "carrier" determinants on an antigen, "line up" an array of small molecules into an immunogenic matrix

The Second Signal Idea

(e) B cell — "second signal" — T cell or macrophage

Two cells come together around a "sandwich" of antigen: the B cell is then induced by a nonspecific signal from the other cell

(f) "second signal" — T cell

Or, the specific receptor from a T cell binds first to the carrier determinants of the antigen and then "signals" the B cell, perhaps by binding to an appropriate receptor for its Fc end on the B cell surface

Fig. 5.11 Possible mechanisms in cell-cell cooperation.

"thymus independent," as we have seen, and also to induce only, or mainly, IgM. It seems that the participation of T cells or their secreted products is a necessary condition for switching B cells from production of IgM to antibody of other classes.

Finally, a teleological point: The purpose of these cell interactions must be to allow better regulation of immune responses. If a single small molecule could stimulate a B cell, anti-self antibody would probably be commonly induced by self-components. A requirement for simultaneous recognition of the self-antigen by T cells would minimize this possibility. As it is, there seems to be a danger that polymeric antigens might bind firmly enough, through multivalency, to

TABLE 5.4
Properties of Cells in the B Line

	Precursor cells ("virgin" immuno-competent cells)	Effector cells (antibody formers)	Memory cells
Function	To generate anti-body forming cells on contact with antigen	Antibody production	As for precursors
Morphology	Small lymphocytes	Varied: plasma cells, basophilic lymphocytes, blasts	Small lymphocytes and large activated cells?
Life history	Probably short life span. Derived from larger, dividing cells, and before that, from hemopoietic stem cells	From immunocompetent small lymphocytes, by proliferation and differentiation; most live only a few days	Develop as part of an expanding clone of antibody forming cells; long life span
Methods of identification	Binding labeled antigen; cloning techniques	Immunofluorescence; microdrops; hemolytic plaque technique	As for precursors
Receptor Ig	IgM only (7–8 S form)	Usually do not bind soluble antigens	IgM + IgD?
Restriction in specificity	Characteristically all make Ig (antibody or receptor) of a single specificity.		
Location	Probably poor recirculating ability	Most localized in lymphoid tissue	Recirculate continuously

stimulate any B cells which have anti-self receptors. Regulating T cells may act in various ways to temper such unwanted reactions. This theme, a product of modern immunological research, will loom larger as we probe more deeply into the subject in subsequent chapters.

5.6 SUMMARY

This chapter first examines some of the properties of *immunocompetent* B cells, lymphocytes which, on stimulation with antigen, can generate antibody forming progeny. These B cells have immunoglobulin *receptor* molecules on their surface which will bind antigen. The cells are *precommitted*, before meeting antigen, to produce receptors of only one specificity, and an antigen selects from a population of lymphocytes a small proportion to whose receptors it can bind.

The development of B cells is briefly discussed: in mammals they arise from stem cells in the fetal liver. In the adult they are produced in the bone marrow.

The cooperative (synergistic) effects of T and B cells in antibody formation have been studied using methods for culturing relatively defined cell populations *in vitro* or in irradiated recipient mice. Two lines of experiment have been described: the "helper" effect of thymus-derived cells on antibody formation by bone marrow-derived cells, and the enhancing activity of T cells primed against a protein antigen on the anti-hapten response made by B cells reacting to hapten coupled to the same protein. Among the possible mechanisms for this cooperation we have considered the formation of matrices of antigen on the B cell surface with possible aggregation ("patching") of its receptors, and the passage of a nonspecific inductive signal from a T cell (or macrophage) to a closely apposed B cell.

FURTHER READING

5.1   Ada, G. L. and Byrt, P. (1969). Specific inactivation of antigen-reactive cells with ^{125}I-labelled antigen. *Nature (London)* **222**, 1291.

5.2   Ada. G. L. and Ey, P. L. (1975). Lymphocyte receptors for antigens. In "The Antigens" (M. Sela, ed.), Vol. III, p. 190. Academic Press, New York.

5.3   Claman, H. N., Chaperon, E. A., and Triplett, R. F. (1966). Immunocompetence of transferred thymus-marrow cell combinations. *J. Immunol.* **97**, 928.

5.4   Cooper M. D. and Lawton, A. R. (1974). The development of the immune system. *Sci. Am.* **231**, 559.

5.5   DeLuca, D., Decker, J., Miller, A., and Sercarz, E. (1974). Antigen binding to lymphoid cells from unimmunized mice: high frequency of beta-galactosidase binding cells at optimal conditions. *Cell. Immunol.* **10**, 1. An alternative view on the specificity of antigen binding by cells.

5.6   Fidler, J. M., Howard, M. C., and Shortman, K. (1976). Antigen-initiated B-lymphocyte differentiation. VIII. Sedimentation velocity and buoyant density characterization of virgin antibody-forming progenitors in the adoptive immune response of unprimed CBA mice to

4-hydroxy-3-iodo-5-nitrophenylacetic acid-polymerized bacterial flagellin antigen. *J. Exp. Med.* **143**, 1220.

5.7 Lefkovits, I. (1972). Induction of antibody-forming cell clones in microcultures. *Eur. J. Immunol.* **2**, 360.

5.8 Marbrook, J. and Haskill, J. S. (1974). The *in vitro* response to sheep erythrocytes by mouse spleen cells: segregation of distinct events leading to antibody formation. *Cell. Immunol.* **13**, 12. Contains a description of a method for "cloning" antibody-forming cells.

5.9 Miller, J. F. A. P. (1962). Effect of neonatal thymectomy on the immunological responsiveness of the mouse. *Proc. R. Soc. London* **B156**, 415.

5.10 Miller, R. G. and Phillips, R. A. (1969). Separation of cells by velocity sedimentation. *J. Cell. Physiol.* **73**, 191.

5.11 Mishell, R. I. and Dutton, R. W. (1967). Immunisation of normal mouse spleen cell suspensions *in vitro*. *Science* **153**, 1004.

5.12 Mitchell, G. F. and Miller, J. F. A. P. (1968). Cell to cell interaction in the immune response. II. The source of hemolysin-forming cells in irradiated mice given bone marrow and thymus or thoracic duct lymphocytes. *J. Exp. Med.* **128**, 821.

5.13 Mitchison, N. A. (1971). The carrier effect in the secondary response to hapten-protein conjugates. I. Measurement of the effect with transferred cells and objections to the local environment hypothesis. *Eur. J. Immunol.* **1**, 10. This and the accompanying article, document the cell cooperation effect in responses to hapten-protein conjugates.

5.14 Moller, G. and Coutinho, A. (1975). Factors influencing activation of B cells in immunity. *Ann. N.Y. Acad. Sci.* **249**, 68. An alternative view on the induction of B cells.

5.15 Pilarski, L. M. and Cunningham, A. J. (1974). The generation of antibody diversity. III. Variation in the specificity of antibody produced within single clones of antibody-forming cells *in vitro*. *Eur. J. Immunol.* **4**, 762.

5.16 Raff, M. C. (1970). Role of thymus-derived lymphocytes in the secondary humoral immune response in mice. *Nature (London)* **226**, 1257.

5.17 Rajewsky, K. V., Schirrmacker, V., Nase, S., and Jerne, N. K. (1969). The requirement of more than one antigenic determinant for immunogenicity. *J. Exp. Med.* **129**, 1131. Cell cooperation shown in a manner slightly different from Mitchison's experiments.

5.18 Shortman, K. (1974). Separation methods for lymphocyte populations. *Contemp. Top. Mol. Immunol.* **3**, 161.

5.19 Vitetta, E. S. and Uhr, J. W. (1975). Immunoglobulin-receptors revisited. *Science* **189**, 964.

5.20 Warner, N. L. (1974). Membrane immunoglobulins and antigen receptors on B and T lymphocytes. *Adv. Immunol.* **19**, 67.

QUESTIONS

5.1 Anti-θ serum (Section 5.3) is usually made by injecting one strain of mice with thymus cells from another. It may also be made by injecting a rabbit with mouse thymus cells. In this case, think about the probable degree of specificity of the rabbit antiserum. What cells in mouse spleen would it affect? How could the serum be made more specific?

5.2 How could you tell whether Ig on the surface of lymphoid cells was being actively produced by those cells or passively acquired (as "cytophilic" antibody—Section 4.2.4)?

5.3 An animal is immunized with an antigen that contains determinants X and Y (antigen XY). It receives a second injection with a different antigen, YZ, and the anti-Z immune response is followed over a period of time. This response occurs more rapidly, and antibody titers are higher than in a typical primary response to YZ in other animals. Why? How could you verify your explanation experimentally?

6

Memory and Tolerance

Immunological memory is the ability to give an *altered* response on second exposure to a specific antigen. The term is usually reserved for occasions when the secondary response is larger than the primary. When challenge produces a depressed response or none at all, a state of *tolerance* is said to exist. Thus, memory and tolerance are opposites. They are both examples of the specific adaptive nature of immune responses, and in fact this adaptivity is a characteristic and defining feature of immune phenomena, even being implied in the word "immune."

6.1 EXAMPLES OF MEMORY

6.1.1 Antibody Titers

In experiments on antibody formation, a state of memory is usually associated with antibody titers which rise more rapidly and to higher levels following a second exposure than they did after the first injection of the antigen (Fig. 1.1).

Variations on this kind of pattern are possible. Sometimes a secondary response is more rapid than a primary, but less total antibody is produced. A lot depends on the antigen, the species of animal immunized, and the interval between primary and secondary injections. This interval should usually be several weeks for best development of a state of memory. As with most immunological phenomena, it is difficult to be certain how a particular individual will behave.

6.1.2 Clinical Immunity

In clinical terms, an individual has memory or is "immune" if he shows increased specific resistance to reinfection with a particular infectious organism. It has been known for thousands of years that this kind of immunity may follow recovery from an initial infection in some diseases. Modern vaccines provide an easier way to acquire such useful memory. The immune system seems to have evolved as a means of resisting recurrent infection with pathogens which were present in the environment. The ability to build up memory, and so resistance, to such organisms was probably even more important than a capacity to give a large primary response. Immunity to infectious disease is further discussed in Chapter 13.

6.1.3 Hypersensitivity

Not all memory is beneficial. We will meet, in Chapter 12, "allergic" or hypersensitive states in which individuals become highly reactive against such environmental antigens as pollens, or food or plant proteins. Similarly, some people when repeatedly injected with a drug, such as penicillin, may become "sensitized" or allergic to it. In other words, they develop immunological memory to the drug, and react rapidly against it in a way which is dangerous. Often, allergic responses are harmful because IgE antibody (Section 3.2) is made. This class of antibody not only combines with antigen but may also cause release of pharmacologically active agents like histamine which produce unwanted effects (Chapter 12).

6.1.4 Changes in Quality of Antibody

Previous experience with an antigen may affect the quality as well as the quantity of a secondary response. The two most important qualitative properties of antibody are its class and its affinity for a particular antigen (see Sections 3.2 and 2.3.3).

With most antigens, the first antibody detected in a primary response is of IgM class, while later a switch occurs to predominantly IgG production. In a typical secondary response, most of the antibody is IgG from the start. A tendency to make large amounts of IgE may result in an allergic memory state as discussed above. Very little is known about the factors which induce production of different antibody classes (but see Section 11.2.2); the presence of a large number of helper T cells seems, however, to favor IgG production over IgM.

The average affinity or antigen binding power (Section 2.3.3) of antibody is usually low at first and increases gradually during the primary response. In a secondary response, the first antibody synthesized is usually of high affinity; cellular reasons for this are discussed below (Section 6.6).

6.1.5 Memory in Other Kinds of Immune Reaction

A state of altered immune responsiveness can be observed even when antibody production is not involved. Thus a second skin graft may be rejected more rapidly than a first from the same donor (Chapter 10). Delayed hypersensitivity

(Chapter 9) is another example of memory, in the T and not the B cell line (see Section 6.4).

6.2 FACTS ABOUT MEMORY

Two points deserve emphasis here: First, memory is *specific* for the antigen encountered. Second, it is often long lasting, a factor which has obvious survival advantage. The maintenance of a state of immunological memory in the body probably depends on persistence of antigen; the life-long immunity which recovery from some virus infections confers may require chronic stimulation by small numbers of virions retained in the body. The long life span of some recirculating memory cells (Section 4.2.3) must also contribute to lasting memory.

6.3 WHAT CAUSES MEMORY?

Figure 6.1 shows the results of an experiment where varying numbers of spleen cells were transferred from normal mice to irradiated recipients, (Section 5.4.1) and stimulated with sheep red blood cell antigen. There were, as usual, a small number (about 100) of "background" antibody plaque forming cells in the spleens of each irradiated mouse whether or not additional spleen cells were transferred. Injection of less than 10^6 cells did not increase this number, but when more than this were transferred an increase in plaques occurred which was proportional to the number of spleen cells injected.

A second group of mice received cells from previously immunized donor mice. Evidently, a particular level of adoptive response could be transferred with about ten times fewer cells, and this difference in activity was maintained over the whole dose range.

This kind of experiment shows two important things. First, memory, in the sense of increased responsiveness, is transferred by a cell suspension. That is, it depends only on the cells themselves, and not on any way in which they are arranged in a primed animal. Second, the proportion of specifically reactive cells is increased by priming (this is currently thought to be the most probable explanation of priming effects, but other possibilities exist, e.g., that inhibitor cells are removed by priming; see also Section 6.8.2).

6.4 PROPERTIES OF THE CELLS RESPONSIBLE FOR MEMORY

In the example cited above it is evident that increased numbers of either specific T or B immunocompetent cells, or both, might have caused the increased

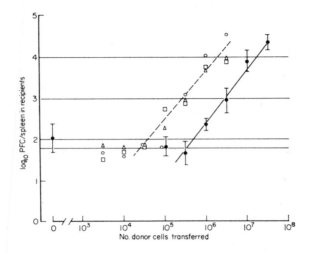

Fig. 6.1 Adoptive transfer of immunological memory. The figure shows the number of antibody–plaque forming cells produced by transfer and challenge of varying numbers of normal or primed spleen cells in irradiated recipient mice (Section 6.3). ●, Normal unprimed donors: △, 3 days; □, 10 days; and ○, 40 days after priming donor mice. Vertical bars show 95% confidence limits of the mean (from Cunningham, Ref. 6.2).

responsiveness of the whole population. Memory, in fact, occurs in both cell lines. The thymus "education" experiment of Miller (Section 5.4.2) was an instance of T memory. The priming of an animal with hapten–protein complexes generates both T and B memory against both hapten and protein (Section 5.4.2); challenge (second injection) with the hapten on a new carrier protein reveals B memory to the hapten.

In the B cell line we can draw a clear distinction between effector cells (antibody formers) and memory cells, which are not themselves making large amounts of antibody, but can be stimulated to generate effector progeny by further contact with antigen. B memory can be transferred by lymphocyte populations from which antibody forming cells have been removed. There are also physiological differences between "virgin" (Section 5.4.1) and "memory" B cells: memory cells have a different distribution of sizes and densities, are longer lived, and many of them recirculate more freely. They have lower electrophoretic mobility than unprimed B cells, and less tendency to stick to glass, which presumably also reflects surface differences. Table 5.4 provides some comparison of the properties of the three members of the B cell line in which we are most interested: the precursor or virgin immunocompetent cell, the antibody former, and the memory cell. Corresponding T cells are dealt with in Chapter 9; similar categories can be recognized although the situation is less clear.

6.5 GENERATION OF MEMORY CELLS

Antigenic stimulation of lymphoid tissue causes proliferation of clones of T and B cells. Within each clone it is probable that some cells become effectors and some memory cells (Fig. 4.14). This has been directly demonstrated in the case of certain B cell clones making anti-hapten antibody with a characteristic pattern of electrophoretic mobility. These clones could be transferred from the animal in which they originated into irradiated recipients, and subsequently retransferred several times; at each transfer new antibody forming cells and B memory cells were made by members of the same clone. Just what causes some cells to become effectors and others memory cells is not clear; by analogy with other inductive events in biology it is probably the nature of their microenvironment that controls this ''decision.'' There is some evidence that B memory cells can develop in the relative absence of T cells, so perhaps it is the availability of T help which controls this aspect of B cell differentiation. T memory cells seem to develop very rapidly after antigenic stimulation, reaching maximum levels in a few days; B memory evolves more slowly (over several weeks).

6.6 "MATURATION OF AFFINITY"

The average affinity of serum antibody for antigen usually rises during an immune response, often by several orders of magnitude; the first antibody produced in a secondary response is characteristically of high affinity. These observations can be readily explained at the cellular level. (Fig. 6.2). The initial (large) dose of antigen stimulates all B cells able to respond to that particular antigen. Most of these release low affinity antibody. As the amount of antigen remaining in the body falls, and becomes *limiting,* so cells with higher affinity receptors have increasingly great survival advantage: these trap antigen and proliferate while low affinity cells are not stimulated. A second dose of antigen encounters a population of B memory cells which are mostly of high affinity, and the antibody produced early in a secondary response reflects this. Thus there is a process of ''evolution'' in the lymphocyte population under the selective influence of antigen (see Chapter 15 and Ref. 6.6 for further discussion).

6.7 TOLERANCE

In Chapter 1, and subsequently, the central dilemma of the immune response has been emphasized: how to respond to any foreign substance, yet not to one's self. A state of specific unresponsiveness, either to self-antigens or to other antigens is called *tolerance.* Research in this area is at a very interesting stage.

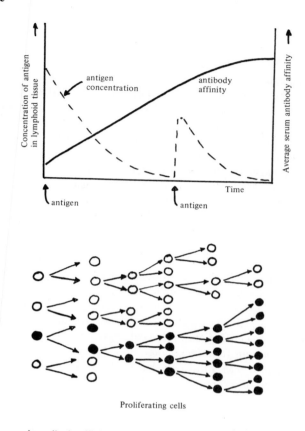

Fig. 6.2 Increase in antibody affinity during an immune response. As antigen concentration falls, cells with high affinity receptors (shown black) "trap" antigen better than low affinity cells; these cells are relatively rare early in the response but proliferate selectively (Section 6.6).

We will look at some basic facts here, and then return to more speculative aspects in Chapter 11. It is important to bear in mind that "tolerance" is an operational definition and simply means that an individual or a population of lymphoid cells responds more poorly to an antigen than it would have done if it had not previously encountered the antigen. No assumptions should be made initially about what is happening to individual cells.

6.7.1 Examples of Tolerant States: Self-Tolerance

An animal does not usually react against its own tissues, a restriction which was called *horror autotoxicus* by Ehrlich, around 1900. When this restriction breaks down we have autoimmune disease, which may take a wide variety of forms, depending on the tissues being reacted against (Chapter 12).

Owen observed, more than 20 years ago, that nonidentical (dizygotic) twin cattle, which shared the same placental circulation, grew up each with red blood cells from the other twin in its blood. If they had not shared a linked circulation during fetal life, these "foreign" red cells would have been rapidly removed by an immune response. From this observation, and from the general fact of self-tolerance, Burnet suggested that any antigens present during early development of an animal would somehow suppress any future response to those antigens when the animal reached maturity. Foreign antigens injected around birth should be treated as "self." Medawar and colleagues demonstrated this experimentally: neonatal injection of X strain cells into Y strain mice was found to decrease the ability of the Y mice to reject an X graft later in life.

6.7.2 Experimentally Induced Tolerance

As a general rule, relatively low molecular weight substances are more *tol-erogenic* (tolerance inducing) than higher molecular weight molecules or particles (which are *immunogenic*). For example, a lot of work on tolerance in mice has been done using gamma-globulin as the *tolerogen*, after it was discovered, by Dresser, that ultracentrifugation removed aggregated material and converted a solution of this protein from *immunogen* to *tolerogen*. Very small molecules (up to several thousand MW) usually have no effect on the immune system, a clue that some kind of receptor cross-linkage may be involved in *tolerogenesis* as it is in induction (Section 5.5). Tolerance is generally easier to induce by injecting neonatal animals rather than adults. Repeated doses of antigen often induce tolerance better than a single dose, perhaps because antigen has to have time to make contact with most of the lymphocytes in the body to which it can bind specifically. There is a great deal of variation in the way individuals respond. Often one or two mice in a batch of ten will be relatively unaffected by a regime which renders the others completely tolerant.

The induction of tolerance in adults by repeated injection of large amounts of antigen was previously called "paralysis," reflecting the belief, now abandoned, that the mechanism was essentially different from neonatally induced tolerance. Very high doses of antigen commonly induce tolerance better than lower doses. However, Mitchison (Ref. 6.5) demonstrated with some antigens (bovine serum albumin was used initially, and others since) that repeated, very low doses ($0.1-1.0$ μg/gm body weight) could induce tolerance in mice. This low zone of tolerance changed to immunity when the dose was increased (Fig. 6.3) and was succeeded by a further *high zone* of tolerance in a dose range of about $1-10$ mg/gm. More recently, it has been found that picogram amounts (1 pg $= 10^{-12}$ gm) of some antigens can induce partial tolerance. ("Partial" here simply means

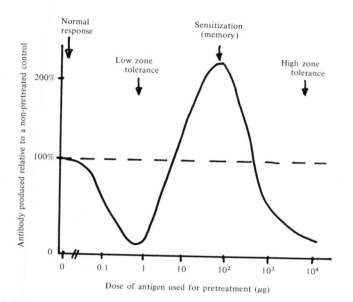

Fig. 6.3 "Zones" of tolerance. Animals are first treated with varying doses of antigen. This may give tolerance or memory. They are then challenged with an immunogenic, standard dose of antigen. The result of various pretreatments is reflected in the size of the secondary response, plotted relative to controls. (After Roitt, Ref. 1.5; adapted from data of Mitchison.)

that the degree of unresponsiveness, while statistically significant, was not dramatic. "Complete" tolerance would imply that no responses could be detected on challenge of tolerant animals; the two differ only in degree.) The reasons for zones of tolerance are still not clear. One hypothesis is that only T cells are affected in the low zone, and both T and B in the high. The phenomenon is not seen with all antigens.

6.7.3 Tolerance in Other Kinds of Immune Reaction

Tolerance, then (like memory), is defined as a *relative* state of unresponsiveness (i.e., low responsiveness) compared with the ability of normal animals to react to the antigen. So we can speak of tolerance in any kind of immune reaction, not only in antibody forming capacity. For example, a state of homograft tolerance may exist in animals injected at birth with cells from another member of the species (Section 6.7.1 and Chapter 10). This would be diagnosed from a relative reluctance of this host animal to reject subsequent grafts of donor strain tissues.

6.8 FACTS ABOUT TOLERANCE

By analogy with the corresponding section on memory (Section 6.2), two important features of immunological tolerance should be mentioned here. First, it is *specific* for the tolerogen: if an antigen caused a tolerance which was general and not specific it would simply be an immunosuppressant drug. Second, it may be long lasting, although it seems that continual presence of the tolerogenic antigen is required if a state of tolerance is to persist.

A beautiful experiment to illustrate this last point was carried out by Triplett in 1962 (Ref. 6.7). He removed the hypophysis (pituitary) from tree frogs, and kept the glands for several weeks (in the dermis of another animal). After this time, each organ was implanted back into the animal from which it was derived. The glands were now rejected: the animals had lost their tolerance to a normal self-component, apparently through not having seen it for some time. In control experiments, half only of the hypophysis was removed, cultured, and reimplanted. These grafts were not rejected. This demonstrated (a) that the organs were not radically altered by culture and (b) that tolerance to this self-component was not lost providing some of it remained in the animal.

6.9 WHAT CAUSES TOLERANCE?

As for memory, this question can be discussed in terms of changes in *individual* cells or changes in *populations* of cells. At the level of individual cells we would like to know whether specifically reactive lymphocytes can be destroyed by antigen when a state of tolerance is induced. While the binding of large amounts of polymeric antigen can sometimes inactivate cells *in vitro,* it is currently uncertain how important such mechanisms are under normal circumstances *in vivo.* In some tolerant states a reduction in numbers of specific antigen binding cells has been reported, in others this has not occurred. It is, in fact, disputable whether such a thing as a "tolerant cell" normally occurs, or whether all tolerance can be attributed to population changes. A tolerant state can, however, be shown (e.g., by the plaque technique) to reflect a definite lack of production of immune effector cells. For example, if an individual is tolerant with respect to its ability to make antibody, there is a significant decrease in the number of antibody forming cells: it is not just a matter of antigen mopping up antibody as it is formed.

In considering tolerance at a second level, the level of cell populations, we should first note that cells from a tolerant animal will often not respond when transferred to, and challenged in, an irradiated recipient. The simplest explanation for this would seem to be that cells reactive to the antigen are actually missing from the population. Burnet considered that self-tolerance was caused by

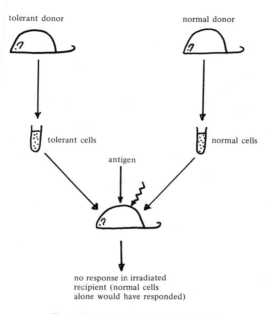

tolerant donor

normal donor

tolerant cells

antigen

normal cells

no response in irradiated
recipient (normal cells
alone would have responded)

Fig. 6.4 Suppressor (active) tolerance.

deletion of clones of cells with self-reactivity (Section 8.3.1). Until a few years ago, this explanation of tolerance was almost universally accepted.

However, this view of tolerance is now questioned as a result of work performed in a number of laboratories. Many examples are now known where cells from a tolerant animal, when mixed with normal cells, will make the whole mixture tolerant (Fig. 6.4). In this case, it is obvious that tolerance is not due to removal of active cells. Rather it seems that specific ''suppressor'' cells have been added. It is currently debated whether self-tolerance can be explained in this way, a question to which we will return in Chapter 11.

6.10 THE CELLS AFFECTED IN TOLERANCE

Obviously, in a system such as antibody formation where at least two interacting components are needed for induction, failure of either component would cause tolerance as an end result. Both T and B cells may be rendered tolerant. A classic experiment demonstrating this is shown in Fig. 6.5 (Weigle, Ref. 6.8). Mice were made tolerant with deaggregated human gamma globulin, then their thymus or bone marrow cells were mixed with normal B or T cells, respectively, and the mixtures tested for their ability to respond to an immunogenic form of the

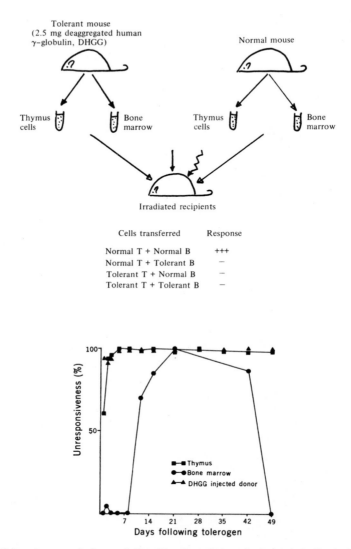

Fig. 6.5 Development of tolerance in T and B cell populations. In the graph the line for "thymus" follows the response of irradiated recipient mice that received an immunogenic form of antigen, normal bone marrow cells, and thymus cells from donor mice injected at various intervals before with tolerogenic antigen. The line for "bone marrow" shows the converse experiment: normal thymus plus tolerant marrow cells. Responses are expressed as a percentage of those given by normal thymus plus normal bone marrow. The line "DHGG injected donor" is the response when both cell types come from tolerant donors (from Chiller, Habicht, and Weigle, Ref. 6.1).

TABLE 6.1
Properties of Memory and Tolerance

	Memory	Tolerance
Examples	Specific resistance to reinfection Higher and faster developing antibody titers Changes in class of antibody Hypersensitivity states Homograft immunity	Self-tolerance Acquired tolerance to foreign antigens; easier to induce neonatally, and to small antigens (high and low zones sometimes seen)
Facts	Specific Long lasting (persistent antigen may be needed)	Specific Long lasting (in presence of antigen)
Probable causes	Increased numbers of specifically reactive cells, T or B or both Changes in nature of specifically reactive cells (e.g., receptor affinity)	Specific deletion of reactive cells? Reversible inactivation, T and/or B cells? Presence of actively suppressive T cells

antigen after transfer to irradiated recipients (Fig. 6.5). Tolerance appeared quickly and persisted in the T cells. The B line became tolerant more slowly and for shorter duration. The interpretation of this work at the time was that T and B cells were deleted, but at different rates. Later developments suggest that other possible interpretations should be considered, i.e., that the tolerance was caused by suppressor T cells, arising in the thymus, and migrating to the bone marrow.

6.11 SUMMARY

Memory and tolerance are opposite sides of the same immunological coin: the ability of lymphoid cell populations to give specifically enhanced or diminished immune responses after initial contact with an antigen. The main properties of these two states are summarized in Table 6.1.

FURTHER READING

6.1 Chiller, J. M., Habicht, G. S., and Weigle, W. O. (1971). Kinetic differences in unresponsiveness of thymus and bone marrow cells. *Science* **171,** 813.

6.2 Cunningham, A. J. (1969). Studies on the cellular basis of immunological memory. *Immunology* **16,** 621.

6.3   Howard J. G. and Mitchison, N. A. (1975). Immunological tolerance. *Prog. Allergy* **18**, 43.

6.4   Miller J. F. A. P. (1973). Immunological memory. *Contemp. Top. Immunobiol.* **2**, 151.

6.5   Mitchison, N. A. (1964). Induction of immunological paralysis in two zones of dosage. *Proc. R. Soc. London* **B161**, 275.

6.6   Siskind, G. W. and Benacerraf, B. (1969). Cell selection by antigen in the immune response. *Adv. Immunol.* **10**, 1. Discusses possible reasons behind the increase in antibody affinity during an immune response.

6.7   Triplett E. L. (1962). On the mechanism of immunologic self-recognition. *J. Immunol.* **89**, 505. A classic paper showing that self-tolerance must be acquired.

6.8   Weigle, W. O. (1973). Immunological unresponsiveness. *Adv. Immunol.* **16**, 61.

QUESTIONS

6.1   After reviewing Section 6.6, predict the effect on the rate of maturation of antibody affinity using (a) very high and (b) very low doses of antigen for primary injection.

6.2   Consider an animal tolerant to an antigen with determinants WXY. Suppose also, that only the T cells reactive against W, X, and Y have been made tolerant and not the B cells. Tolerance may now be broken, i.e., antibody induced against this first antigen, by injecting a cross-reacting antigen XYZ. How might this breaking of tolerance occur? Against which determinants of the first antigen would the antibody elicited by XYZ be directed?

6.3   In an experiment on the cloning of specific antibody forming cells *in vitro*, culture of 5×10^5 normal mouse spleen cells in a Marbrook raft for 3 days produced specific, anti-sheep erythrocyte plaque forming cells in 10 of the 36 culture wells (Section 5.4.1 and Fig. 5.5). However, when the same number of cells were cultured from a mouse previously immunized with sheep erythrocytes, every well in the raft contained specific plaque forming cells. Why?

Antibody Diversity: Its Genetic Basis

We have seen that an individual can make antibody against an almost unlimited number of foreign antigens without reacting against himself. Just how many different antibodies can be made is unknown, but it is almost certainly more than a million (Chapter 2). In this chapter we will briefly discuss the genetic basis for this great diversity, without worrying unduly (until Chapter 8) about how anti-self reactivity is avoided. The main questions to be considered are:

1. Is there a unique gene coding for each different antibody polypeptide chain made (the "instruction versus selection" debate);

2. If so, are all of these genes present in the germline (zygote) DNA or are the majority created during the life of the individual (the "germline versus somatic mutation" dilemma)?

7.1 INSTRUCTION VERSUS SELECTION

There are, in theory, two basic ways in which lymphoid cells might produce antibody molecules with combining sites adapted to any antigen which is encountered. The first is by *instruction:* the antigen acts as a template around which the antibody molecule folds itself to form a complementary structure. The second is *selection* by antigen of one of a vast range of preexisting antibodies, followed by a stimulus to produce more of the same antibody. Roitt in "Essential Immunology" (Ref. 1.5) gives an analogy to illustrate this difference. Old-fashioned tailors were *instructed* by a client to make a suit to measure: the client acted as the template around which the cloth was molded. The modern chain-store tailor makes 10^4 suits, one of which is supposed to fit any specific purchaser, and clients *select* a preformed article. On the face of it, instruction is simpler. We

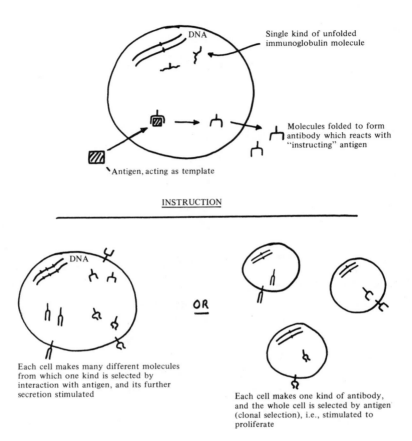

Fig. 7.1 Instruction and selection theories for generation of antibody diversity.

could make do with one or very few genes whose products could adopt many shapes.

The history of this debate is interesting, with waxing and waning support for both sides. Ehrlich, around 1900, was the first to speculate seriously on generation of diversity. He was a selectionist. In his view, cells had preformed antibodies (side chains) which combined with antigen and somehow stimulated production of more antibody of the same specificity. However, with the realization (Landsteiner) that the body could produce antibodies against many artificial haptens and discriminate between them, the idea emerged that antigen might directly instruct cells (Haurowitz, Pauling). (It should be remembered that at this time, around 1920–1940, almost nothing was known about how proteins are synthesized.) Instructionist theories reigned for many years. Then in 1955 Jerne revived discussions of selection, and in 1959 Burnet published his book on the clonal selection theory (Section 8.3.1). Today, it is almost unanimously agreed that each antibody molecule is coded for by a separate gene, and thus that selection of preformed antibody molecules by antigen takes place. Some of the reasons for this belief are summarized below:

1. Modern ideas on protein synthesis (DNA → RNA → protein) make instruction (protein → protein) difficult to accept. Antibody synthesis is found experimentally to occur in the same way as synthesis of other proteins.

2. Allied to this is the fact that the primary structure of a protein is now known to determine its tertiary configuration. A great variety of primary structures exist. This argues against the idea that antibody with a single amino acid sequence is folded to fit many different antigens. More recently it has been found that "unfolded" (partially denatured) antibody molecules may refold and regain some combining activity in the absence of antigen. Thus the tertiary structure of antibody does not depend on the presence of antigen.

3. Antibody forming cells appear to have little or no antigen inside them, as would be required by the template theory. This was shown by Nossal and collaborators using highly radiolabeled antigen and autoradiography of single antibody forming cells.

4. If instruction occurs, each immunocompetent cell ought to be "multipotent," i.e., in the case of B cells, able to make any antibody depending on what antigen gets inside. By contrast, selective theories predict that cells are preordained to make one particular antibody before encountering antigen. The first experimental evidence for selection came when Nossal showed that, in animals immunized with two antigens, any one cell makes only one antibody. On reflection, however, we can see that this is not unequivocal proof of selection: each cell might be multipotent, but directed to the synthesis of one particular antibody after its first contact with antigen. Final vindication of Burnet's ideas came as the great sequence diversity among antibodies was appreciated, and, at the cellular level, from demonstrations that immunocompetent cells were committed to making one antibody specificity before "seeing" antigen (Section 5.2.2).

7.2 GERMLINE VERSUS SOMATIC MUTATION

Since antibody production obeys the normal laws of protein synthesis, it follows that each different antibody polypeptide chain must come, via messenger RNA, from a gene in the DNA. The main debate about the *genetic* basis of antibody diversity currently centers on whether all possible V genes are in the

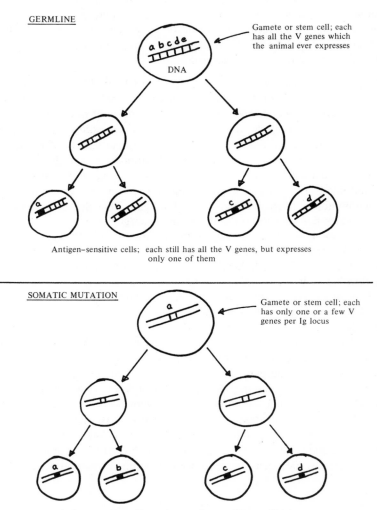

Fig. 7.2 Germline and somatic mutation theories for generation of diversity.

germline (that is, in the haploid, gamete DNA) or whether only a few genes are inherited, with new genes being rapidly created during the life of an individual by some random process such as mutation or recombination in the V gene parts of the DNA. Various hypothetical mechanisms have been proposed by means of which a few genes could give rise to many. We will briefly consider two possibilities here: sequential point mutation and a "gene interaction" model.

While "somatic mutation" is often loosely used to include any kind of somatic genetic event which generates new V genes, in its original form this theory proposes that, from an initial very small array of genes, new ones emerge through a series of single base changes (Fig. 7.3). The rate of mutation may or

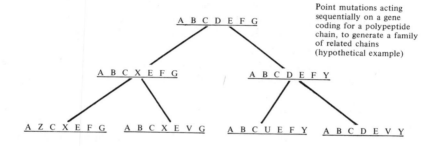

Point mutations acting sequentially on a gene coding for a polypeptide chain, to generate a family of related chains (hypothetical example)

Amino acids in hypervariable regions at positions indicated (counting from NH₂ terminus)

		1st			2nd			3rd	
λ chains		26	30		48	50	55	92	95
1 – 12	All identical, = basic sequence	Ser	Ser		Ile	Gly	Ala	Tyr	His
13	1 Substitution	Asn							
14	1 Substitution				Leu				
15	1 Substitution						Val		
16	1 Substitution							Cys	
17	2 Substitutions	Thr	Gly						
18	4 Substitutions	Asn			Asn				Arg

Fig. 7.3 Generation of families of V genes by point mutation. The top diagram shows the principle. The lower table is an actual example: 18 mouse V_λ chains have been sequenced. Twelve are identical; four more differ from this basal pattern by one amino acid (explicable as a single base change); the remaining two have undergone 2 and 4 base changes. All substitutions are in hypervariable regions of the molecule. (After Cohn, Ref. 7.3, based on the work of Weigert *et al.*)

may not be higher than at other loci, but an important element of the model is that cells expressing mutated receptors are subject to strong selective pressures; if the mutation has occurred in the hypervariable part of the V region (Section 3.4), and has favorably affected the ability of the cell to bind to an antigen, the cell will be selectively stimulated by that antigen; if the mutation was in other parts of the V gene or in the C gene, it will not be selected for. We would thus expect that most of the observed variation should be in the hypervariable regions. This has been confirmed in mouse λ chains which make up only about 3% of mouse Ig light chains (Fig. 7.3). There are only 18 mouse V_λ sequences known: twelve are identical, four vary from this by a single amino acid (each explicable as one base change), and two more vary by two and three amino acids from the parental sequence. All substitutions are in hypervariable regions. This pattern is obviously consistent with a point mutation process to generate V gene diversity. Note, however, that the sequences alone do not tell us over what time period this mutation occurred: it could be during somatic life (i.e., the life span of the individual), only the basic V gene being inherited, or it could have taken place during evolutionary time, each individual inheriting all (seven) different V genes.

Several models have been proposed based on recombinational events between a small number of initial V genes (e.g., Gally and Edelman, Ref. 3.10). An interesting recent one is that outlined by Wu and Kabat and developed by Capra and Kindt (Fig. 7.4 and Ref. 7.2). Each Ig polypeptide chain comes from at least three interacting genes, one for the C region, one for the relatively invariant or

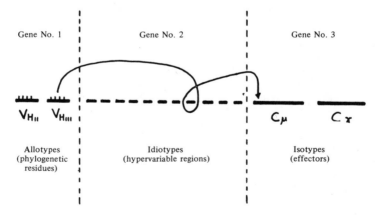

Fig. 7.4 Hypothetical genes involved in the synthesis of human IgG chains. The arrow indicates selection of one gene from each group prior to synthesis of an H chain. A complete DNA sequence might be "put together," prior to transcription, by a process of recombination, translocation, or episomal insertion. (From Capra and Kindt, Ref. 7.2.)

framework part of the V region, and one or more for the hypervariable regions. Possibly 50–100 of these last genes, plus a very few for framework V regions, would be sufficient. The genes would link up by a translocation, episomal insertion or recombination process, as shown in the figure. This kind of model can explain the finding referred to in Section 3.6: antibody V regions from two unrelated individuals with identical hypervariable sequences.

7.2.1 Numbers of Genes Required

Obviously the germline theory is the more complicated. The human haploid genome contains only enough DNA for about 10^7 V genes, which looks awkward for the germline theory if an individual can make a million or more different antibodies. However, its proponents nimbly suggest that 1000 V_L and 1000 V_H genes would be sufficient to produce 10^6 (1000 × 1000) $V_L V_H$ combinations, each antibody combining site depending on a contribution from both chains. This assumes that the majority of random L–H combinations produce functional antibody, which is unproved although probably reasonable.

As discussed earlier (Section 3.7), actual "counting" of V genes by molecular hybridization seems to be indicating that there are very few of these genes in the DNA of each cell.

7.2.2 Genetic Drift

If there are very large numbers of inherited antibody genes, how are they all retained, generation after generation, when only a small fraction are used by any one animal? For example, how have genes coding for antibody to artificial antigens such as arsanilic acid or dinitrophenol been preserved throughout evolution when they presumably have no survival advantage? This seems a serious objection to germline theory. Its defendants usually reply that antibody against arsanilic acid may, for example, cross-react strongly with common pathogens; the ability to react against foreign antigens is a by-product of the retention of other antibody V genes important for survival.

7.2.3 V Region Allotypes

The discovery of genetic markers (allotypes, Section 3.3) in rabbit V genes also appears to favor the mutational theory. The same characteristic marker (small sequence of amino acids) is found in the V regions of *all* of the (thousands?) of antibodies of different specificities produced by one Ig family in a rabbit. According to the germline theory, the marker must be present in all of the corresponding genes, which are linked to one another in the DNA. However, because of the extensive crossing-over which occurs during gametogenesis, we

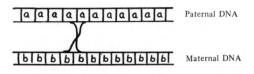

Fig. 7.5 The V region allotype dilemma (Section 7.2.3). If the germline theory is correct, there must be many different V genes in the DNA, each of the same allotype. This allotype homogeneity should be disrupted by meiotic crossing-over in the V region of the DNA in animals which have received different allotypes from each parent.

would expect many of these genes to be quickly replaced, during evolution, by alleles bearing a different marker (Fig. 7.5). Mutation would also tend to destroy the pattern. By contrast, if there were only one germline V gene in an Ig family, which gave rise to hundreds more by mutation, then all derivatives of that gene would bear the marker. V region allotypes are clearly much easier to explain by somatic mutation.

However, two recent groups of findings conspire to weaken the advantage of the mutational view in explaining this point. First, since the discovery of V region subgroups (Section 3.6) it has become necessary to postulate more than one V gene per locus; if there are three V_κ subgroups then there must, it is said, be at least three V_κ germline genes. Second, it now seems that the rabbit "allotypes" are not allotypes at all! Individual rabbits may produce at least three of them under some conditions. The apparent simple Mendelian inheritance of the allotypes may have been brought about by meiotic segregation of some regulatory gene(s) controlling expression of different V region allotypes, all of which were present in the DNA of all individuals. Similar anomalies are beginning to be reported in expression of Ig allotypes in mice and men (the question is enormously complex; a good starting point for further reading is Williamson's recent review, Ref. 3.17).

7.2.4 Species-Specific Residues

A similar argument, which we will not discuss in detail, concerns the amino acid patterns common to V regions of one species but different in all V regions of other closely related species. The difficulty for germline theory arises when we consider the DNA of the common ancestral species. If this had many V genes, why is it that all the genes in one descendant line of animals adopted one particular pattern, while another descendant species all retained another and different characteristic V region structure?

In attempting to answer this and the previous point, proponents of the germline theory generally invoke special mechanisms of DNA behavior, for example, that crossing-over is prevented in some way within the long block of V genes, as mentioned above, and that "expansion" and "contraction" of these regions of the genome (from many genes down to a few and back again) may occur over short intervals of evolutionary time (Ref. 3.12).

7.2.5 How Are Mutant Cells Produced and Selected?

This point forms the spearhead of the attack by germline theorists on somatic mutationalists. According to the latter, a very large number of mutant cells must be made during development of an individual, and useful ones selected. These mutants might, for example, be made by *hypermutation* at V loci (Section 3.6). The weakness of this idea, in the absence of direct evidence for it, is that it is apparently a novel mechanism. Germline proponents can fairly point out that if hypermutation can be invoked, so equally can prevention of crossing-over! We will return to the question of rates of mutation at antibody loci in the next chapter. We should also note that models can be put forward assuming a normal mutation rate in V genes but with very intensive selective pressures favoring mutants.

7.3 WHICH IS CORRECT—GERMLINE OR SOMATIC MUTATION?

Antibody diversity seems to be, overall, much more easily explained by the somatic mutation theory. The author may have betrayed a hint of bias in his earlier remarks, and he will now admit to an unashamed belief in somatic variation as the means of creating antibody diversity. Nevertheless many immunologists still support germline ideas, which can be pursued in Refs. 3.12 and 7.8. An opinion may be offered as to why the germline theory still has its adherents. There seem to be two main reasons:

1. Until the recent hybridization work, most of the arguments have been indirect and based on inferences from myeloma protein sequences. The *time* dimension, which is the essence of the problem, really, has been largely ignored. We want to know, not that V regions fall into subgroups which can be represented as a tree (Section 3.6), but how fast and how reproducibly this process can occur.

2. There has often been a failure to realize how organisms cope with an

unpredictable environment (see Chapter 1). The evolutionary process depends on producing random variants, which are selected for if advantageous. It is reasonable to suppose that this basic biological mechanism applies to antibodies (and the cells which produce them) as much as to whole animals. Superficially, it may seem simpler to have all the genes in the germline, but in practice this is too great a load to carry, and too inflexible in the face of unexpected new antigenic challenge (see also Chapter 15).

7.4 SUMMARY

This chapter has examined the two major questions concerning the genetic basis of antibody variability:

1. Do cells produce one or a few multipurpose antibodies which adopt their final shape by folding around an antigen template? Or is each antibody coded for by a unique gene? The former *instructionist* theory, once widely held, has been abandoned in favor of the latter alternative, since it is now known that different antibodies have different primary amino acid structures. Cells spontaneously make one kind of antibody, and are *selected* (and stimulated) by antigen which binds to these antibody receptors.

2. Are all the genes for all possible antibodies inherited in the gamete DNA (*germline theory*), or are a few V genes inherited, and a vast array of new ones generated by *somatic mutation* among lymphoid cells? This debate continues, although the evidence we have cited favors the somatic mutation theory.

FURTHER READING

7.1   Burnet, F. M. (1959). "The Clonal Selection Theory of Acquired Immunity." Cambridge University Press, London. The classic exposition of clonal selection.

7.2   Capra, J. D. and Kindt, T. J. (1975). Antibody diversity: can more than one gene encode each variable region? *Immunogenetics* **1**, 417. Expounds the model shown in Fig. 7.4.

7.3   Cohn, M. (1974). A rationale for ordering the data on antibody diversification. *Prog. Immunol.* **2**, 261. Inferences from antibody sequences by a somatic mutationalist.

7.4   Gally, J. A. and Edelman, G. M. (1970). Somatic translocation of antibody genes. *Nature (London)* **227**, 341. (Discusses some possible recombination mechanisms also.)

7.5   Haurowitz, F. (1973). The problem of antibody diversity. Immunodifferentiation versus somatic mutation. *Immunochemistry,* **10**, 775. A recent statement by a pioneer of the instructive theory.

7.6   Jerne, N. J. (1955). The natural selection theory of antibody formation. *Proc. Nat. Acad. Sci. (U.S.A.)* **41**, 849.

7.7   Lederburg, J. (1959). Genes and antibodies. *Science* **129**, 1649.

7.8   Wigzell, H. (1973). Antibody diversity: is it all coded for by the germ line genes? *Scand. J. Immunol.* **2**, 199. Argues for the germline theory.

QUESTIONS

7.1 List the main arguments for germline and somatic mutation theories on the origin of immunological diversity.

7.2 If you were a proponent of the instructive theory of antibody diversity, how would you account for tolerance to self-components?

7.3 The observed variation in antibody sequences is much greater in V than in C regions (Chapter 3). Assuming somatic mutation as the means of generating antibody diversity, is it necessarily true that the rate of mutation in V genes is higher than that in C genes?

8

Development of the Immune Repertoire and Self-Tolerance in the Individual

As we have seen, every individual has a wide variety of immunocompetent cells, each bearing on its surface an antibody receptor molecule of a particular specificity. This array of lymphocytes is sufficiently diverse to ensure that most antigens will combine with the antibody of at least some of the cells. Yet the thousands of different self-antigens will not stimulate any of them. In this chapter we briefly consider how this diverse yet selective *repertoire* of immunocompetent cells is built up. In Chapter 11 there is some additional discussion of self-tolerance, and of the subtle regulatory mechanisms controlling which clones are allowed to expand after antigenic stimulation.

8.1 ALLELIC EXCLUSION

In the last chapter we saw that antibody diversity reflects V gene diversity. Instructionist ideas are no longer tenable. There is still no consensus as to whether all these antibody genes are inherited or created anew in each individual. Nevertheless, it is clear that, however many antibody genes it may possess, an immunocompetent cell makes receptors of only one specificity, and that what happens to a cell depends on the impact of antigens on these receptors. If the receptor antibody reacts specifically against the antigens of a pathogenic environmental microorganism, that cell is likely to be stimulated to proliferate; if it reacts against a self-component, the cell must be suppressed in some way.

At this point the discerning reader might raise the following objection: "A diploid cell has two genes at each locus. So in a heterozygote, if the cell was making μ and κ chains there might well be two μ chains with different V regions, and two different κ chains. Four different antibody combining sites would be possible by random combination of the H and L chains. If the cell expressed all four receptors, one might react against a foreign antigen and another against a self-component.'' This possibility is eliminated because of *allelic exclusion,* a unique and important property of immunocomponent cells.

Consider a mouse heterozygous at one of its C gene loci: assume it has *a* and *b* alleles coding for a and b allotypes (Section 3.3) of that protein. Now we would expect Ig of both a and b types in the serum, and this is found. However, when we look at individual Ig producing cells, for example, by staining them with both anti-a and anti-b fluorescent antibody (using two different fluorescent dyes), a remarkable fact emerges. *Each cell produces only one allotype,* a or b, but not both. The animal contains a mixture of both kinds of cell. This allelic exclusion—only one of two alleles at an antibody locus expressed per cell—is unique among mammalian diploid cells. It is not known how the inactivation of one allele occurs. For all other proteins (e.g., hemoglobin), both alleles in the cell make a product, although in heterozygotes the two products may be different, one being defective in some cases, or nonfunctional, and the other phenotypically dominant. (The only other similar example known, where one allele, or in this case one whole chromosome, is suppressed, is the X chromosome in females. Here the maternal or paternal X chromosome is inactivated randomly, forming a Barr body, so every female is a mosaic of two different kinds of cell, one with an active maternal X, the other with a paternal X.)

It appears then that the restriction of immunocompetent cells is ''complete'': each produces only one kind of L and one H chain at any one time. That is, it produces antibody with one specificity of combining site, one class (defined by H chain type) and one allotype. It seems likely that this mechanism has evolved to allow selection of a cell, by antigen, on the basis of its single homogeneous Ig product, without the ambiguity of having to decide between several different receptors (Ref. 1.8).

8.2 SELF-TOLERANCE IS ACQUIRED

Is it conceivable that an animal is *genetically* incapable of reacting immunologically against itself? That it has no cells with anti-self receptors because it has no genes for anti-self antibody? This notion still appears in the literature from time to time. However, it can be simply shown to be impossible. An ''A'' animal has the capacity to react against all foreign antigens including those of other strains, ''B,'' of the same species. Thus it must have genes that code for ''anti-B,'' and B likewise has ''anti-A'' genes. The offspring (A $\times$ B) of an A and a B parent must inherit at least some of these genes from each parent: this hybrid now has the genetic potential to produce anti-self-reactive cells and so to destroy itself. Since it does not do this, it follows that this potential is suppressed in some way, i.e., self-tolerance is acquired or learned. This is a basic and vitally important property of the immune system.

At this stage it may be worth referring back to Triplett's experiment (Ref. 6.7) on removing part of the pituitary gland from frogs (see Section 6.8); the animals gradually lost their tolerance to this self-component, again showing that normal individuals have the ability to react against their own antigens, but that provided these are constantly present, self-reactivity is usually prevented in some way. The fact that self-tolerance must be actively learned is also nicely shown in *tetraparental* mice, animals made by fusing together early blastocysts from two different embryos. These animals develop normally to adulthood although they contain cells of both kinds; a viable adult can be made by fusing "A" and "B" blastocysts when each of these strains would normally react violently against antigens of the other. In the tetraparental state they learn to coexist.

8.3 VIEWS ON GENERATION OF DIVERSITY

We are now able to look at the views of several authors on the development of the immune repertoire. The main things we want to know are (1) when, how fast, and under what conditions the great array of different lymphocytes arises; and (2) how self-tolerance is assured, i.e., how those lymphocytes with anti-self reactivity are inactivated. These questions are *epigenetic,* that is, they are concerned with levels of organization "higher" than the DNA, with the way cells interact, during development with one another and with their environment. The questions exist regardless of the underlying genetic basis of diversity, and are not solved by knowing the genetic mechanisms. As in much of immunology, we will be discussing theories framed at the cellular level (Section 4.1).

8.3.1 Burnet: Clonal Selection

Against a prevailing belief in instruction, Burnet wrote his clonal selection theory, published in 1959 (Ref. 7.1). His argument was the Darwinian one that lymphoid cells generate diversity randomly, and are selected by antigen on the basis of "fitness," or strength of binding, in this case. He was the first to stress that the unit selected must be the whole cell with its homogeneous receptors, and he predicted "one cell–one antibody" (Section 4.6.3). Prior to this, it had been vaguely assumed by those few immunologists interested in selection that antigen might select one of many different antibodies displayed by a single cell, and thus encourage further production of that particular product. Burnet cut through this fog, and pointed out that immunological memory could be established by selective proliferation of stimulated clones (Fig. 8.1). The major elements of this idea

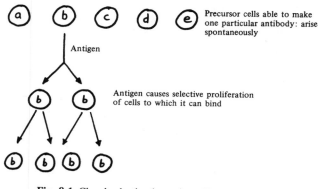

Fig. 8.1 Clonal selection by antigen (Burnet, Ref. 7.1).

are now universally accepted, and clonal selection stands as probably the most important single theory in the field.

Burnet also assumed that the genetic basis for antibody diversity was hypermutation in the V genes of immunocompetent cells early in the development of an individual. This process was essentially complete soon after birth. Lymphoid cells were assumed to be especially sensitive at this early stage of the individual's development: if an antigen bound to them, the cells were destroyed rather than stimulated. Normally the only antigens accessible to lymphocytes before birth would be self-components; thus, anti-self-reactive cells were purged from the population. If foreign antigens were administered early enough (e.g., just after birth), they too would induce tolerance in the same way. This explanation of self-tolerance was accepted for many years. However, it seems unlikely to be entirely correct for three main reasons: (1) it is now known that cells in an adult animal can be made tolerant, that is, there is no critical period for inducing tolerance; (2) a state of tolerance can be induced by mechanisms other than destroying specifically reactive cells, for example, by suppression of a specific response, as discussed in Section 6.8.2; (3) when an organ is removed, immune reactivity against it appears (Section 6.8). Thus anti-self reactive cells exist or can be produced in adult animals. This is discussed further in Section 11.2.3.

8.3.2 Jerne: Negative Selection Theory

Niels Jerne has made many important theoretical and other contributions to immunology. Around 1955 he discussed selectionist ideas. In 1974, he published a "network theory" (Ref. 11.15) for control of immune responses, which we will examine in Chapter 11, and in 1971 he proposed a scheme for simultaneous development of the immune repertoire and self-tolerance (Ref. 8.6). This last idea is a difficult one, which may be easier to understand after reading Chapter 10. It starts with the observation that a high proportion of an individual's lymphocytes is capable of reacting against *allogeneic* tissues, that is against cells from other individuals of the same species but of a different inbred strain (see Chapter 10). Why these reactive lymphocytes should exist was unknown. Jerne suggested that in an embryo, all lymphocytes initially possess an inherited reactivity against the histocompatibility antigens (see Chapter 10) of the same species. Perhaps 90% of these are potentially reactive against those histocompatibility antigens of the species *not* present in the individual; these cells persist into adulthood. The remainder are potentially reactive against the antigens possessed by the individual himself: these can not survive unless their antibody receptors change due to a mutation in the corresponding gene, a mutation which reduces their ability to react against self. Such mutants are not killed, but proliferate. Additional cycles of mutation in such cells can increase their survival advantage (Fig. 8.2), and these mutants ultimately serve as the repertoire of cells able to react against foreign antigens.

This theory is ingenious, but has some drawbacks, one being that it now seems that there are other ways of explaining the apparently high levels of alloreactive cells (Chapter 10). Another is that it is difficult to explain how self-antigens and the inherited anti-self antibody genes could evolve in parallel: mutations would break up the correspondence (Ref. 8.1).

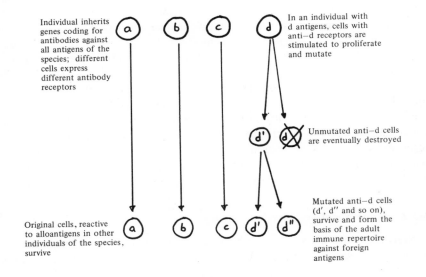

Fig. 8.2 Somatic evolution of allogeneic reactivity and ability to respond to foreign antigens (Jerne, Ref. 8.6).

8.3.3 Associative Recognition

Bretscher and Cohn (Ref. 8.3) have attempted to explain how the "decision" is made as to whether a cell will be stimulated or inactivated (tolerized) in terms of a simple "switch" at the surface of the lymphocyte. Basically, their theory proposes that if antigen by itself comes into contact with a cell, that cell is "paralyzed" ("one-hit" → tolerance). If a second determinant on the antigen is simultaneously bound by another antibody, then the cell is induced and not paralyzed ("associative recognition"). This second antibody would probably be on a T cell, or secreted by a T cell and bound to the surface of a macrophage (Fig. 8.3; and see also Section 5.5.3).

This idea leads fairly naturally to an explanation for self-tolerance: it is assumed that all self-antigens are present before the immune system matures. Antigen-reactive cells arise, not all together, but in a gradual way. If they bind an antigen in their environment (normally a self-antigen), they are immediately paralyzed by the "one-hit" mechanism. If they are not reactive to self but to a foreign antigen X, they survive. So anti-self reactive cells never have time to accumulate, being made tolerant one by one as they arise. Immunocompetent cells with receptors for foreign antigens, on the other hand, are not destroyed, and appear in large numbers. If, now, antigen X is given to an adult animal, there are enough anti-X cells around to ensure that specific T and B cells will simultaneously recognize the same antigen molecules. Therefore, induction, not tolerance, results.

Note that there is no *intrinsic* difference between self- and foreign antigens, but that there is a difference in the times at which they are present in the animal. Self-antigens are *continuously* present, and usually from an early age. It is this feature, common to all self-antigens, which Bretscher and Cohn have emphasized in their analysis.

This theory, besides explaining self-tolerance, also can account for most other major immunological phenomena, such as cell–cell cooperation (Section 5.5), zones of tolerance (Section 6.7.2), and the relative thymus independence of

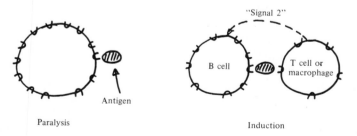

Fig. 8.3 Associative recognition (Bretscher and Conn, Ref. 8.3).

polymeric antigens (Section 5.5.2). Many immunologists consider that the mechanisms for tolerance/induction discrimination must be more complex than Bretscher and Cohn propose, and it is true that their theory does not encompass the modern work on suppressor mechanisms in tolerance. Nevertheless, it stands as a considerable intellectual feat, the reduction of an immensely complex body of data down to a simply digital ''on-off'' switch at the cellular level, and is a good example of the kind of unifying theory which must be sought in many scientific disciplines. A clear discussion of the theory is given by Bretscher (Ref. 8.2).

8.3.4 Germline

A perfectly logical theory for generation of diversity (GOD) and self-tolerance can be constructed on the assumption that all antibody genes are in the germline. Rather than the progressive enlargement of the repertoire of immunocompetent cells by somatic variation during development, it is expected that different lymphocytes simply express only one of the vast array of V genes which they carry at each Ig locus. Methods for suppressing or deleting anti-self-reactivity could be the same as for somatic theories.

8.3.5 Generation of Diversity After Antigenic Stimulation

It has usually been assumed that all members of a clone of immunocompetent cells proliferating after antigenic stimulation continue to produce exactly the same antibody. However, it has recently been shown by Dr. L. M. Pilarski and the author that rapid variation can take place within developing clones. The simplest demonstration of this was to culture single antibody forming cells *in vitro* (for 2 days) until they divided to give up to twelve offspring. In a high proportion of these small clones, different members produced antibodies with slightly different specificities. Other experiments have shown that this also occurs naturally, *in vivo*. (This work is reviewed in Ref. 8.4.)

These new findings lead to a very different view of the generation of diversity. Instead of cell specificities being inherited or created spontaneously, relatively few are made in the young animal. As the animal begins to make contact with environmental antigens, certain clones are stimulated, and ''throw off'' a number of slightly different variants, some of which are selected by antigen. It makes sense that the repertoire should evolve in this way, in the directions required to meet the stimuli of a particular environment (Fig. 8.4). A corollary of the model is that anti-self-reactive variants must be produced in large numbers during normal immune responses. This leads to a prediction that self-tolerance is assured by some means of continuous suppression of self-reactive cells, rather than by their deletion (further discussed in Chapter 11). No contradiction of clonal

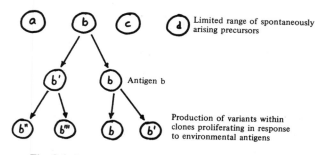

Fig. 8.4 Generation of diversity after antigenic stimulation.

selection is implied: cells are precommitted, before antigen, to making one kind of antibody receptor, but as they proliferate random variants appear at a high rate and are available for selection by antigen. The process is a Darwinian evolutionary one, but enormously accelerated (see also Chapter 15).

This theory, being very new, is not yet widely accepted. A major stumbling block has been the apparent need for hypervariation in stimulated clones, which would require a unique genetic mechanism. This should not discredit the theory since the immune system is itself unique, and is already known to employ unusual mechanisms, allelic exclusion (Section 8.2) and translocation (Section 3.5).

8.4 ONTOGENY OF THE IMMUNE REPERTOIRE

It should be possible to measure experimentally just when the diverse repertoire of immunocompetent cells arises. A lot of work has been done in this area without any consensus having as yet been reached. There are four main possibilities, all of which have their adherents:

1. Essentially all of the receptor specificities that an individual will ever make are represented among immunocompetent cells early in development.

2. There is a gradual "programmed" (i.e., regular) expression of different receptor specificities during development, and up to, say, young adulthood. That is, mice always start making antibody one on day 16 of gestation, antibody two on day 17, etc. Such a model seems to require a germline inheritance of V genes.

3. Gradual enlargement of the repertoire, but by entirely random processes, giving different repertoires in different individuals.

4. Much of the diversity among immunocompetent cells is generated within proliferating clones of antigen-stimulated cells (Section 8.3.5).

Arguments for and against each view are too involved to consider here. References 8.4 and 3.5 are possible starting points for additional reading.

TABLE 8.1
Theories on Generation of Diversity and Development of Tolerance in an Individual

	Mechanism of GOD	Time of production of new antigenic reactivities	How self-tolerance is achieved	How increased reactivity to foreign antigens is achieved
Germline	All genes inherited	Evolutionary time	Not specified: some kind of suppression of self-reactivity	Clonal expansion of pre-existing cells (selected by antigen)
Burnet: clonal selection theory	Somatic hyper-mutation	During early development	Deletion of self-reactive clones neonatally	As above
Jerne: negative selection	Somatic mutation of self-reactive cells	As above	Death of unmutated self-reactive cells	Selection of mutants of self-reactive cells for nonreactivity to self, followed by clonal selection by antigen
Associative recognition (Bretscher/Cohn)	Continual production of new mutants	Throughout life	Deletion of self-reactive cells, one by one as they arise	Induction of cells if antigen is recognized by two cells at once
Generation of diversity *after* antigen (Cunningham)	Probably hyper-mutation	Throughout life	Active suppression	Variation and selection within clones responding to antigen

8.5 GENERAL REMARKS

Perhaps the main lesson to be gained from these conflicting theories is that the immune system is a *learning* system. Lymphocytes learn from their environment. No one seriously questions that self-tolerance is learned, although whether by deletion or suppression of self-reactive cells is not clear. Also everyone accepts Burnet's idea of the basis of immunological memory: selection and differential expansion of different clones. It is when we come to the initial way in which the diversity is expressed that disagreements appear.

On one extreme the germline theorists argue that immune diversity is "learned" just like any other biological diversity, by the slow process of mutation and natural selection during evolutionary time. In the middle are the somatic mutationalists who see rapid, random creation of all possible antibody specificities during ontogeny, useful ones being selected. As Cohn puts it: "an antibody is a theory which a cell makes about its environment." At the other extreme is the newest view: relatively few specificities are spontaneously created, but environmental antigen stimulates some clones, which then rapidly produce a number of random variants, around a central theme as it were. There is less waste. The changing environment has the "information" which directs the development of an individual's immune repertoire along those lines which will be most useful to it, but without violating Darwinian principles.

8.6 SUMMARY

First the phenomenon of allelic exclusion is described. By this mechanism, immunocompetent cells transcribe only one light and one heavy chain gene, and thus can be selected by antigen on the basis of a single antibody receptor product. Next, it is argued that self-tolerance must be learned, not inherited. Finally, several views are given on the generation of diversity and acquisition of self-tolerance by individuals (Table 8.1). These have in common that the immune repertoire must, to some extent, be learned by interaction with the environment.

FURTHER READING

8.1   Bodmer, W. F. (1972). Evolutionary significance of the HL-A system. *Nature (London)* **237**, 139. Includes a criticism of the Jerne hypothesis on generation of the immune repertoire.

8.2   Bretscher, P. A. (1972). The control of humoral and associative antibody synthesis. *Transplant. Rev.* **11**, 217. A clear discussion of the Bretscher/Cohn theory, Section 8.3.3.

8.3   Bretscher, P. and Cohn. M. (1970). A theory of self-nonself discrimination. *Science* **169**, 1042.

8.4   Cunningham, A. J. (1976). Evolution in microcosm: the rapid somatic diversification of lymphocytes. *Cold Spring Harbor Symp. Quant. Biol.* **41,** in press. Also published in: *Ann. Immunol. (Paris)* **127C,** 531.

8.5   Jerne, N. K. (1971). What precedes clonal selection? *In* "Ontogeny of Acquired Immunity," p. 1. Elsevier, Amsterdam. A discussion of the probable size of the repertoire of immunocompetent cells.

8.6   Jerne, N. K. (1971). The somatic generation of immune recognition. *Eur. J. Immunol.* **1,** 1. A discussion of the "negative selection theory" outlined in Section 8.3.2.

QUESTIONS

8.1   You might like to convince yourself of the importance of allelic exclusion in immunocompetent cells by doing the following calculation. Assume allelic exclusion does not occur and that each cell makes receptors of four different specificities. Assume also that 3 out of 4 possible antibody receptors can react with self-antigens and only 1 out of every 4 does not. What proportion of cells would have only receptors with specificities for foreign antigens?

8.2   Compare the predictions made by germline and somatic mutation theories on the number of possible different antibodies that (a) an individual, and (b) a species, can make.

8.3   Heavily irradiated mice (Section 8.4.1) can be prevented from dying by injection of bone marrow cells, since bone marrow contains precursor cells which restore their hemopoietic and lymphoid systems. Bone marrow is taken from mice X and Y, representatives of two antigenically different strains each of whose lymphocytes will react fiercely against antigens of the other strain. The cells are mixed and injected into a lethally irradiated recipient mouse (don't worry, until after reading Chapter 10, about the genetic constitution of this recipient). What will happen to this mouse, and why?

9

More about T Cells

Until now we have mainly discussed antibodies and the B cells which synthesize them. This brought us to a point where we could examine the fundamental problem of immunology, the generation of diversity and the development of a population of cells responsive to foreign antigens but tolerant of self. In the past, B cells have been much more thoroughly studied than T cells, mainly because their product, antibody, could be so easily collected, characterized, and used as a label to identify the cells producing it and their precursors. However, the other arm of the immune system, T cell function, is equally important, and has become the subject of much of the current research effort in cellular immunology. Several features of T cells make them more difficult to study than B cells: they have very diverse functions; the nature of their antigen-specific receptors has proved difficult to demonstrate and is still controversial; and there are no simple, single cell tests as yet generally available for identifying individual, specific effector cells.

We will look first at the generation of immunocompetent T cells in the thymus, then at the properties of these cells, and, later, discuss some of the effector functions of T cells.

9.1 DIFFERENTIATION OF T CELLS

The thymus is a large, white, bilobed organ situated in the upper chest. Histologically it consists of a sessile matrix of specialized epithelial cells packed with large numbers of lymphocytes. In most species the thymus is well developed at birth, grows in size until puberty, and then involutes (shrinks) during adult life.

9.1.1 Evidence for Immunological Activity of the Thymus

R. A. Good and F. M. Burnet speculated that the thymus was in some way important for the development of immune responses, since the gland was absent or abnormal in some immunological deficiency diseases. Then, in 1962, Miller showed experimentally that removal of the thymus from newborn mice (neonatal *thymectomy*) drastically reduced the ability of these animals to make immune responses later in life. The thymectomized mice had smaller numbers of circulating lymphocytes than normal mice, usually did not reject grafts from other strains of mice (Chapter 10), and produced less antibody to many antigens. They also developed a wasting syndrome called "runt disease," which could be attributed to inability to combat infection, since neonatally thymectomized mice reared under germfree conditions remained healthy.

These observations strongly suggested that many of the circulating immunocompetent lymphocytes were produced (by division from other cells) within the thymus. That this is so can be confirmed in the following way. When a mouse is heavily irradiated, to kill all dividing cells in the thymus and elsewhere, and then injected with bone marrow cells bearing some marker foreign to the host, within 1 to 2 weeks T cells with the donor marker begin to appear in the recirculating pool and peripheral lymphoid tissue of the recipient. When the irradiated recipient is thymectomized this reconstitution of peripheral T cells does not occur.

After years of controversy, during much of which time it was thought that thymus lymphocytes were derived from fixed "reticular" cells in the thymus, it has become accepted that the precursors of T cells are migratory, basophilic, hemopoietic stem cells. These issue from the yolk sac initially in fetal life, and from bone marrow in adults, and settle in small numbers in the thymus.

Removal of the thymus from adult animals has little immediate effect on their ability to respond immunologically in any way, although in mice, antibody forming capacity may be diminished several months after the operation. It appears that most of the "seeding" of thymus lymphocytes to the periphery occurs early in development. The adult animal may rely mainly, for its immune responsiveness, on long-lived, recirculating, memory lymphocytes.

When θ-negative (Section 5.3) cells from bone marrow or fetal liver are incubated for 2 hours *in vitro* with concentrated extracts from thymus, a proportion of these cells express surface antigens characteristic of T lymphocytes (θ and Ly antigens, see below). This and other evidence on the restoration of some immune function to thymectomized animals by thymus extracts (Ref. 9.6) has led to the suggestion that the thymus makes a hormone "thymosin," in addition to its function as an organ where T lymphocytes proliferate and differentiate. It is still not clear, however, whether effective concentrations of such thymic humoral factors exist outside the organ itself.

9.1.2 Development of T cells within the Thymus

Topical application of radioactive nucleosides to the capsule of the thymus labels large dividing cells in the cortex or outer part; after 24 hours labeled small and medium cells appear in the inner medulla, and by 3–5 days following the initial labeling, most of the heavily labeled cells are medullary small lymphocytes. This implies that medullary lymphocytes arise by division from large cortical cells. Other experimental attempts to work out developmental pathways include physical fractionation of cells by size, density or electrophoretic mobility (Section 5.2.5), and treatment with antisera to surface antigens, in particular, with complement and anti-θ serum (Section 5.3) at various dilutions; cells with "high θ" content are lysed by small amounts of the serum. A further useful finding has been that hydrocortisone selectively destroys cortical thymic cells leaving behind the medullary small lymphocytes which can then be shown to be responsible for most of the mature effector (e.g., helper) activity of the whole population.

Such observations have led to the developmental scheme for thymus lymphocyte shown in Fig. 9.1. This is certainly oversimplified: e.g., Shortman (Ref.

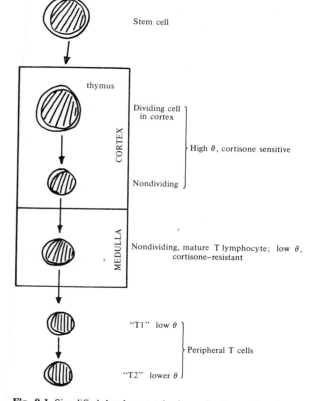

Fig. 9.1 Simplified developmental scheme for thymus lymphocytes.

9.13) has proposed a more complex scheme. Two additional points are most important: (a) there is constant rapid proliferation of lymphocytes in the thymus, and (b) most of the lymphocytes generated there never leave the organ, but die and disintegrate. Why this should be so has intrigued many workers; perhaps the most interesting idea is that the majority of T cells react with self-antigens while still in the thymus and are destroyed, while those which do not react with self escape into the circulating pool. However, there is no evidence for this.

A possible sequence of events in T cells leaving the thymus is also shown in Fig. 9.1. The emerging cells ("T1") seem to be short-lived, nonrecirculating, rapidly dividing lymphocytes which "home" preferentially to fixed lymphoid tissues, where, perhaps on contact with antigen, they generate long-lived recirculating "T2" cells with less θ antigen on their surfaces.

T cells in mice constitute about 35–40% of splenic lymphocytes, 65–70% of those in lymph nodes and blood, and 85–90% of the lymphocytes in the thoracic duct.

9.1.3 Distinguishing T from B, and Subclasses of T Cells

It is often important to be able to assess the relative proportions of T and B cells in a lymphoid population, or to separate one class of lymphocyte from the other. Table 9.1 shows the main techniques available. Some further explanatory comments listed below may be helpful:

TABLE 9.1
Distinguishing B and T Cells

Property or marker	T	B
1. Anatomy	In thymus	In bone marrow (precursor cells in fetal liver)
2. Genetic deficiency; thymus-less "nude" mice	No T cells	Normal B cells
3. Surface Ig	− or ±	+ +
4. Nylon wool columns	Pass through	Adhere
5. Other physical separation techniques	Size, density, electrophoretic mobility	Size, density, electrophoretic mobility
6. Antilymphocyte serum	Preferentially affects recirculating T cells	Little affected
7. Surface θ antigen	+ +	
8. Mitogens		
PHA	+ (stimulates)	− (Does not stimulate)
Con A (monomeric)	+	−
LPS	−	+
PWM	+	+
9. Other surface alloantigens	Ly, TL (see Table 9.2)	MBLA

1. We have already seen (Chapters 5 and 6) how thymus and bone marrow may be used as relatively pure sources of T and B cells.

2. The ''nude'' gene in mice is a recessive mutation which in homozygous animals leads to congenital absence of a thymus (and also to hairlessness—hence the name). Such mice have been useful in demonstrating the limited immune responsiveness of B cells without T cells. They do not reject tissue grafts (Chapter 10), but make relatively small amounts of mainly IgM antibody to some antigens.

3. As we will see below, T cells are not affected by anti-Ig antisera plus complement (at least in most laboratories!). This treatment is commonly used to remove B cells from a mixed population. Anti-Ig may also be coupled to a solid support, usually on a chromatographic column, and used to filter B cells selectively from a population of lymphocytes passed through the column.

4. B cells stick to Nylon wool under certain conditions, while T cells do not. This forms the basis of a simple column procedure for removing B cells (they cannot be recovered from the Nylon wool; T cells only are obtained).

5. Of other direct physical separation techniques, electrophoresis apparently gives the cleanest fractionation of T and B cells (Ref. 5.18).

6. Antilymphocyte serum is made by injecting lymphocytes from one species of animal into another (thymocytes are often used as the antigen, although the terms ''antithymocyte'' and ''antilymphocyte'' are generally used interchangeably). Such sera preferentially deplete recirculating T cells when injected back into animals of the species donating the lymphocytes. They slow down rejection of grafts (Chapter 10), and are used therapeutically in humans for this purpose.

7. We have already discussed the θ or Thy-1 antigen (Section 5.3) which is present on T, but not B, cells of mice. Two allelic forms of θ are known; e.g., the T cells of CBA strain mice act as an antigen in AKR mice, and vice versa. An antiserum selective for T cells can be made by repeatedly immunizing AKR strain mice, for example, with CBA strain T cells (Fig. 9.2). Incubation of a

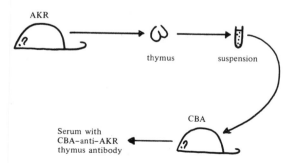

Fig. 9.2 Preparation of anti-θ serum.

mixed cell population with anti-θ serum and complement will remove T cells selectively. The T cells in a tissue can also be revealed with anti-θ serum to which a fluorescent tag has been attached. Other cell surface antigens present on T and not B cells are the TL (thymocyte leukemia antigen, found only on immature T cells) and some of the Ly antigens (see below). Antisera against them are made in a similar way to anti-θ serum. The "MBLA" (mouse bone marrow lymphocyte) antigen is a similar entity, but is found on B not T cells (it has not been widely used). The surface antigens provide a very simple way of removing or identifying lymphocyte subpopulations.

8. Various substances of plant origin (phytohemagglutinin, PHA; concanavalin A, Con A; pokeweed mitogen, PWM) or from bacteria (lipopolysaccharide, LPS) have the power to stimulate proliferation in subpopulations of lymphocytes, as shown in Table 9.1. These and other mitogens stimulate all lymphocytes of one kind, regardless of their immune receptor specificities. For example, LPS induces the formation of antibody of many different specificities in cultured B lymphocytes, and is, therefore, sometimes called a "polyclonal activator" (some mitogens stimulate only one apparent subclass of cells within T or B categories, however).

It has recently become possible to subdivide T lymphocytes into three smaller categories using sera prepared against alleles of the "Ly" series of differentiation antigens. *Ly-1* is a locus on chromosome 19 in mice, and *Ly-2* and *Ly-3* are closely linked loci on the sixth chromosome. An antiserum against Ly-1 antigen would be made in the same way as described above for anti-θ: by immunization of mice that have one allelic form of the antigen with thymocytes from another strain, carrying a different allele. It appears that immature thymic cells, expressing all three of these Ly antigens (Ly-1$^+$,2$^+$,3$^+$) give rise to two lines of progeny Ly-1$^+$ and Ly-2$^+$,3$^+$. Different kinds of effector T cells, which we will discuss later in the chapter, fall into these two groups (Table 9.2). Further subdivision of T cells on the basis of surface antigens seem inevitable.

9.2 IMMUNE RECEPTORS ON T CELLS

While there is reasonable agreement about B cell receptors (Section 5.2) the pursuit of corresponding receptors for antigen on T cells has led to a quagmire of conflicting results. Two groups claim to have isolated 8S IgM immunoglobulin from the surface of T cells; other workers using similar techniques have not been able to find these molecules. Binding of antigen by a small proportion of T cells has been recorded by some groups and denied by others, although it now seems fairly clear that specific binding can occur, particularly if the antigens are in high concentration, or are of large size, e.g., aggregated proteins or erythrocytes. Where antigen binding has been shown, attempts have usually been made to

TABLE 9.2
Functions and Ly Phenotypes of Various Subsets of T Cells[a]

T Cell type	Activity	Ly antigens on surface	
		Ly-1	Ly-2, -3
Immature cells	Precursor of effector T cells	+	+
Regulation			
Helper cells	Regulate antibody production by B cells, and also induction of	+	−
Suppressor cells[b]	other T cells	−	+
Cellular immunity			
Cytotoxic T cells[c]	Kill target cells	−	+
Liberators of lymphokines	Cause delayed-type hypersensitivity reactions	+	−

[a] This table is likely to become obsolete very quickly (compiled late 1976).

[b] Ly phenotypes of helper and suppressor cells have been studied mainly in T cells which affect antibody formation. Those which regulate the activity of other T cells may have different properties, and, in fact, T cells suppressing delayed hypersensitivity reactions have recently been found to have the same Ly antigen pattern as helper cells (they may *be* helper cells).

[c] It seems that cytotoxic and suppressor cells differ in other surface antigens, although they have the same Ly phenotype.

inhibit it with anti-Ig sera, sometimes with positive and sometimes with negative results. Binding seems to be detected more readily if the T cells, after exposure to antigen, are treated with a histological fixative such as glutaraldehyde. The mystery is deepened by reports that a high proportion of thymus cells (up to 2% from fetal animals) will, in some cases, bind certain enzyme and bacterial antigens.

There are a number of possible reasons for the difficulties experienced in demonstrating antigen binding by T cells, some of which are shown in Fig. 9.3; the receptors may be less numerous than on B cells, of lower affinity, "buried" in the membrane, or rapidly shed. Interpretation of experiments is complicated by the fact that some T cells are known to be capable of taking up B cell Ig "cytophilically" (Section 4.2.4), that is, the Ig sticks to the surface of the cell by its Fc end. However, two kinds of observation support the view that T cells synthesize their own receptors. First, in the hands of some workers, receptors can be capped and removed with anti-Ig (Section 5.2.4); the cells appear to recover specific antigen binding power if incubated *in vitro* for several hours. Second, "suicide" experiments (Section 5.2.2) have been reported, removing specific helper T cell activity with highly radiolabeled antigens. Such destruction of a

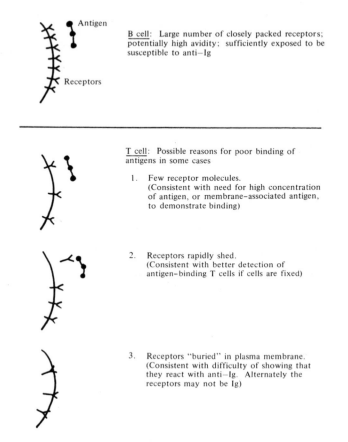

Fig. 9.3 Possible reasons for the difficulty of demonstrating antigen binding by T cells.

specific function indicates that the antigen binding cells are biologically important. It is difficult (although not impossible) to see how cytophilic antibody could be preferentially bound to a small fraction only of a T cell population. Recent reports show that, in contrast to B cells, T cells bind antigen better at 37°C than at lower temperatures, perhaps indicating that the binding is an active process which involves more than simple combination of antigen with relatively static receptors.

9.2.1 Sharing of Idiotypes of B and T Cell Receptors

There is some exciting recent work which provides further information on the nature of T cell receptors. Before proceeding further, however, we need to define the term *idiotype* (Fig. 9.4). Every Ig V region has, as well as antibody activity, an antigenicity which stems from its own unique structure. Antibodies can be made against the V regions (and particularly against the hypervariable parts) of other antibodies. The individual antigenicity of the V region of an Ig molecule is called its idiotype. It should be distinguished from allotype (Section 3.3) which is common to many immunoglobulin molecules with different combining activities.

We can now outline work done by Ramseier and Lindenmann, and by Binz and Wigzell. Animals of one inbred strain (Section 10.4.1) can make antibody against the antigens of a different inbred strain of the same species. "X" makes antibodies to "Y" (Fig. 9.5). The idiotypes of these X-anti-Y antibodies are apparently similar from one X individual to another. An F1 hybrid animal, "X × Y," made by crossing an X individual with a Y, will not normally make antibody against itself, being self-tolerant (Section 8.2). However, if we inject into it some X-anti-Y antibody, the *idiotypes* of this will be recognized as foreign, and will provoke specific anti-idiotypic (anti-antibody) response, i.e., anti-(X-anti-Y). This anti-idiotype serum will, of course, react specifically with the idiotypes that provoked it. It is a useful reagent which can be used to test a variety of ideas. For example, Binz and Wigzell, working with rats, wanted to know whether T cells had on their surface antibody of the same idiotype as that made by B cells. This

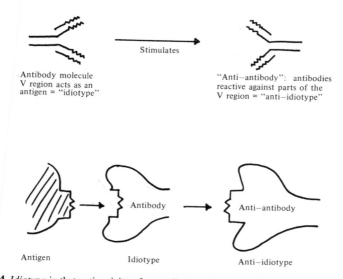

Fig. 9.4 *Idiotype* is that antigenicity of an antibody which stems from its own unique structure. Therefore, an anti-antibody directed against parts of the V region of another antibody molecule is "anti-idiotype," i.e., it has specificity for the idiotype of the initial antibody. The lower part of the figure shows diagrammatically how anti-idiotype can mimic the original antigenic determinant which provoked the first round of antibody formation.

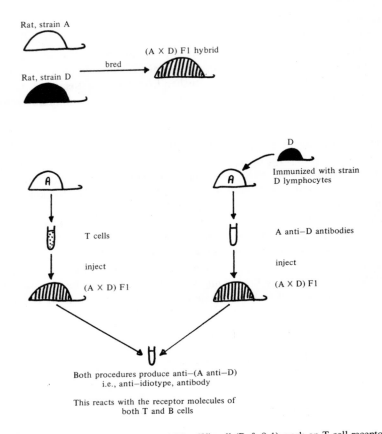

Rat, strain A

Rat, strain D

bred

(A × D) F1 hybrid

D

Immunized with strain
D lymphocytes

A

A

T cells

A anti–D antibodies

inject

inject

(A × D) F1

(A × D) F1

Both procedures produce anti–(A anti–D)
i.e., anti–idiotype, antibody

This reacts with the receptor molecules of
both T and B cells

Fig. 9.5 The Ramseier–Lindenmann and Binz-Wigzell (Ref. 9.1) work on T cell receptors.

was shown to be so since their anti-idiotype serum reacted with T cells and specifically inhibited only those T cells which had X-anti-Y specificity. In other words, specific X-anti-Y T cells carried on their surface receptor molecules with the same idiotype as specific X-anti-Y antibody produced by B cells. Converse experiments, immmunizing F1 animals with X-strain T cells, induced anti-idiotype antibody with similar properties (Fig. 9.5).

This work, and the concept of idiotype, are often difficult to grasp at first, although they should become clearer after reading Chapters 10 and 11. The main point here is that T cell and B cell receptors seem to share idiotypes, which implies that they have the same Ig V regions. It is not yet known exactly what kinds of T cell have these receptors. Using anti-idiotype serum to purify secreted T cell receptors, it has been very recently claimed that T cell receptors are polypeptide chains of molecular weight approximately 75,000, which may normally be associated as dimers. They are not, however, affected by conventional anti-Ig sera. The simplest view at the moment is that T cell receptors have a new class of heavy chain, i.e., that they use the same V regions as are found in B cell immunoglobulins but a different C region, and that they seem to have no light chains at all. These views are borne out by an equally exciting (but even more complex!) independent series of experiments by Eichmann and Rajewsky, which involve the use of anti-idiotype antibody to prime mouse T and B cells for immune responses to streptococcal antigens: these will not be described here. Both lines of work can be pursued further from Ref. 9.4. The perceptive reader may predict that, in any antibody response, the new idiotypes generated will provoke anti-idiotype production. This may indeed be the case, as is discussed further in Section 11.2.2.

9.3 MEMORY AND TOLERANCE IN T CELLS

We have seen, in Chapters 5 and 6, that T helper cells can show memory and tolerance. Thymus-derived cells were "educated" to perform a helper function in Miller's experiments (Section 5.4.2). Priming with a protein induces an anti-θ sensitive population of cells which help B cells respond to a hapten (Section 5.4.3). Tolerance in the T population was demonstrated in Weigle's experiments (Section 6.10; Fig. 6.5) where thymus cells from tolerant mice could no longer induce normal bone marrow cells to make antibody. Similarly, T cell tolerance may be inferred from "hapten–carrier" type experiments, following an experimental design also introduced by Weigle. This may be easier to understand if it is explained in abstract terms rather than by exactly describing the experiments. If tolerance is induced to antigen X, and then the tolerant animal is challenged with X covalently coupled to another antigen, Y, it will now make an immune response. The anti-Y part of the response should be normal (but see Section 11.2.1). If anti-X antibody is made, this is said to mean that B cells of this specificity were unaffected, and that only the T cells had been rendered tolerant to X (deleted), cooperation having occurred with T cells specific for the new, Y, part of the antigen, that is, anti-Y T cells helped anti-X B cells (Fig. 11.2).

It seems, then, that T cells, like B cells, are arranged in clones of different specificities. This clonal distribution is implied by the specificity of T memory and tolerance, and borne out by the antigen and anti-idiotype binding experiments described earlier. If all T cells had the same specificity, obviously T memory and tolerance would not be specific. Memory and tolerance can also be shown for the other T effector functions which we will discuss in the next sections.

There is some evidence for cooperation between subsets of T cells in the induction of effector T cells. It also appears that the initial morphological changes which a T cell undergoes after induction may be the same as for B cells: transformation and proliferation giving rise to larger basophilic cells, which can then divide further to produce more small lymphocytes. Overall, however, much less is known about the clonal development of T cells than of B cells; we have, for example, no good estimates of the sizes attainable by effector T cell clones. Our ignorance is largely attributable to the lack of technical methods for detecting individual active T cells.

9.4 T CELL EFFECTOR FUNCTIONS

While the B cell appears to have only one task, making antibody, the T cell is much more versatile. Its activities can be grouped into two major divisions (Table 9.2):

1. The regulation of immune reactions by other cells. We have discussed how T cells help the induction of B cells, and have also encountered the idea that T cells can suppress B cell responses. It now seems probable that regulation by T cells is important in all immune reactions, including those made by other T cells.

2. Direct interactions between T cells and antigen that do not involve B cells or antibody. This latter kind of activity has historically been called "cellular immunity" because it can be transferred from one animal to another only with cells and not with serum (Section 9.4.2). It is further divisible into two different categories (Table 9.2): those effects produced by T cells which, on contact with specific antigen, liberate *nonspecific* pharmacologically active materials (Sections 9.4.1–9.4.3), and those effects produced by "cytotoxic" T cells which directly attack antigens on the surface of foreign cells (Sections 9.4.4 and 9.4.5).

An additional point should be noted here: B cells liberate specific molecules which circulate around the body. T cells, by contrast, often exert their effects through specific molecules which remain attached to their surface. In some cases, they release nonspecific products which have local inflammatory action. In performing their helper and suppressor functions, T cells may release specific effector molecules, as we will discuss in Chapter 11, but it is probable that these act only in the immediate vicinity of the cell producing them.

9.4.1 Cellular Immunity: The Tuberculin Reaction

When the tubercle bacillus (*Mycobacterium*) infects an animal, it lodges in tissues like the lung and multiplies extensively, often living inside macrophages. This activity promotes a local inflammatory reaction by the host (Section 4.3).

Some of the bacterial antigen reaches the lymph nodes draining the area, and there is clonal expansion of T cells able to react with the antigen in the nodes.

When a small amount of antigen from tubercle bacilli is injected under the skin of an animal or man, a characteristic reaction occurs if, and only if, the subject has previously become sensitized to the antigen. A red lump appears, which grows in size for about 24 hours then fades over the next 1-2 days. Histologically, the skin in this area is heavily infiltrated with lymphocytes and monocytes. This is called the tuberculin reaction and the kind of sensitivity to antigen which results in slow local reactions like this is called *delayed hypersensitivity* (we will look at the mechanisms shortly). Such reactions can be contrasted with the much more rapid *immediate sensitivity* mediated by antibody (Section 12.2.2).

While infection with tuberculosis is the prototype of this kind of reaction, delayed-type hypersensitivity develops against many infectious disease organisms (Chapter 13), and can be induced to many, perhaps all, antigens if they are administered in particular ways, e.g., emulsified in certain adjuvants (Section 4.3), or in very small amounts, or as complexes with antibody. Some simple chemical substances, like picryl chloride, if painted on the skin, will combine with self-proteins and then induce delayed hypersensitivity to themselves.

9.4.2 Transfer of Cellular Immunity with Cells, not Serum

Earlier (Section 2.4) we saw that a state of humoral or antibody dependent immunity could be passively acquired by the simple process of transferring serum from immune to normal animals. However, immunity to tuberculosis, and a state of delayed hypersensitivity to other antigens can not be transferred in this way. It is necessary to transfer lymphoid cells (Fig. 9.6), as was first shown by Chase in 1942. Guinea pigs which received sufficient numbers of lymphoid cells from other individuals immune to tuberculosis were found to acquire delayed-type hypersensitivity, that is, they made a positive skin test, when challenged, and were more resistant to the disease. Similarly, the ability to reject tissue grafts (Chapter 10) can be transferred with cells and not usually with serum.

Nossal, in his book "Antibodies and Immunity" (Ref. 1.4), presents an interesting analogy to illustrate the fundamental distinction between humoral and cell-mediated branches of the immune system. Warfare involves both long range and hand-to-hand fighting. Antibodies are like bullets: once they have left their point of origin, they are effective by themselves. Where antibodies are responsible for an immune reaction the serum containing them will confer immunity, for a short time, on another individual (although memory *cells,* the rifle bearing soldiers must be transferred for prolonged adoptive immunity). The hand-to-hand fighters are those T cells which are involved in reactions classified as cell-mediated immunity. They do not liberate antibodies or other stable, long-range specific molecules. The cells themselves, bearing some kind of specific surface molecules, are the effector units.

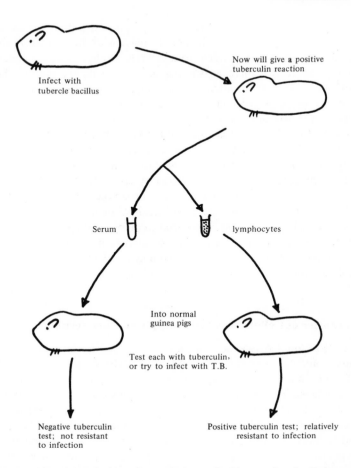

Infect with
tubercle bacillus

Now will give a positive
tuberculin reaction

Serum

lymphocytes

Into normal
guinea pigs

Test each with tuberculin,
or try to infect with T.B.

Negative tuberculin
test; not resistant
to infection

Positive tuberculin test; relatively
resistant to infection

Fig. 9.6 Immunity to tuberculosis can be passively acquired by transfer of cells but not serum from an immune donor.

9.4.3 Generation and Function of T Cells Active in Cell-Mediated Immunity

On appropriate stimulation by antigen within lymphoid tissue, certain kinds of immunocompetent T cell are stimulated to undergo clonal proliferation, with the generation of T cells of phenotype Ly-1^+,2^- (Table 9.2). These are variously known as "delayed-type hypersensitivity" or "DTH" T cells, or simply as "sensitized" T cells. They appear within a few days, but the state of sensitization which they confer on an animal may last for months.

When a second injection of antigen is given, these sensitized, recirculating T cells become trapped at sites where antigen is held, e.g., in foci of infection. There they bind antigen and then release pharmacologically active factors, often called *lymphokines*. These are a heterogeneous group of nonspecific proteins with molecular weights ranging from 35,000 to 150,000. They have diverse properties: some lymphokines will aggregate macrophages, while others attract polymorphs and monocytes to their site of release. A further important function of this class of substances is the *activation* of macrophages, inducing them to phagocytize and destroy foreign antigens more vigorously. *In vitro* assays for lymphokine release exist, e.g., the immobilization of macrophages may be observed when specific T cells are treated with the antigen to which they were previously sensitized. *In vivo* there is a local inflammatory response, of the kind exemplified by the tuberculin reaction, with infiltration of the site by mononuclear cells. These reactions can be regarded as a primitive kind of defense mechanism which confers some degree of protection by ''walling off'' an infected area from the rest of the body.

The *specificity* of these delayed-type hypersensitivity reactions deserves further comment. The initial contact with antigen generates T cells sensitive to that antigen. Second contact with the same antigen is necessary to cause release of lymphokines, but once released, the lymphokine action is not antigen-specific, e.g., an immune reaction to the tubercle bacillus may protect an animal against simultaneous challenge with *Brucella* organisms.

Delayed-type hypersensitivity reactions are as strong in animals without B cells (e.g., in bursectomized chickens) as in normal animals. They are important in tuberculosis, lepromatous leprosy, some fungal and parasite diseases, mycoplasmoses, and some viral diseases.

9.4.4 Cytotoxic T Cells

If an animal is sensitized against an antigen on the surface of a foreign cell, then active T cells may develop which will kill this "target" cell *in vivo* or *in vitro*. These *cytotoxic* T cells are distinct from the kind which liberate lymphokines, e.g., they have a different pattern of Ly antigens (Table 9.2). Exactly what conditions favor the generation of one kind of sensitized effector T cell rather than the other is not as yet clear. Killing by cytotoxic T cells involves direct attachment to the target cell via specific receptors; the target cell is lysed; complement is not required for the reaction; the cytotoxic cell is not destroyed and may move on and kill additional targets. Cytotoxic T cell activity is commonly measured *in vitro* by lysis of target cells and release of radioactively labeled cytoplasmic constituents into the supernatant medium (Fig. 9.8).

T effector cells of this kind develop with specificities against antigens on cells in grafted tissues (Chapter 10), and they are important in the rejection of such grafts. Cytotoxic T cells are also generated within animals infected with certain

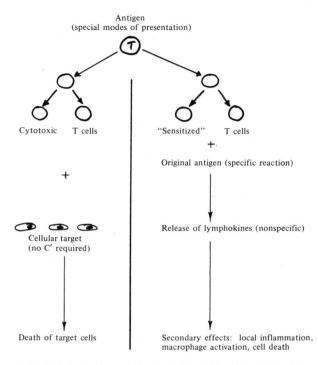

Fig. 9.7 Comparison of "cytotoxic" and "sensitized" T cells.

viruses, e.g., poxviruses and paramyxoviruses. These "killer" T cells react against viral antigens on the surface of infected cells, and by killing such targets may limit the spread of the virus. Similar cytotoxic cells can be induced to react against haptens coupled to the surface of cells.

9.4.5 Restricted Recognition by T Cells?

A recent observation on the behavior of cytotoxic T cells has created a great deal of interest. When such cells are obtained from a mouse of strain X infected with virus, they will kill infected target cells of the X strain but not cells of another strain of mice, Y, infected with the same virus (Blanden, Doherty, Zinkernagel). Similar rules apply to hapten-coupled target cells. This kind of *restriction* had been previously observed in helper T cells; helper cells from an animal of strain X primed against a protein antigen would cooperate with B cells of the same strain, but not with B cells of strain Y (Kindred and Shreffler and Katz and Benacerraf). These obviously related phenomena have stimulated a lot of speculation; the simplest explanation would seem to be that T cells of either

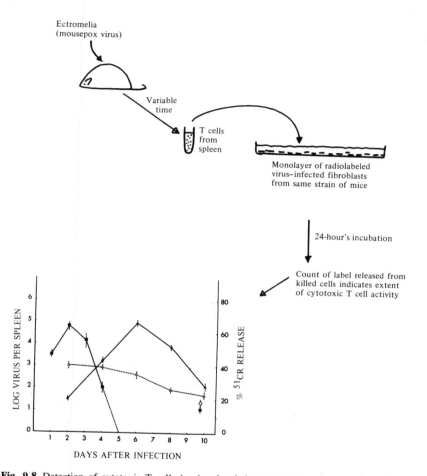

Fig. 9.8 Detection of cytotoxic T cells *in vitro* by their power to lyse target cells and release radioactive cytoplasmic label. The left-hand curve (■———■) follows the growth and decline of ectromelia virus in the spleen (expressed as log₁₀ viral plaque forming units per spleen). The curve ▲———▲ follows the specific T cell cytotoxic activity generated in the spleen at various times after infection, and tested on target cells infected with virus. The curve △ - - - △ is a control showing relatively low cytotoxicity of the same splenic T cells on *uninfected* fibroblasts (from Blanden and Gardner, Ref. 9.2).

helper or cytotoxic varieties become sensitized, not against a protein alone or a virus alone, but against the foreign antigen associated in some sort of complex together with normal cell surface antigens. Thus cytotoxic T cells from animal X infected with virus have receptors specific for "(X plus virus)." This topic can be pursued in Refs. 9.4, 9.5, and 9.12.

Among the spin-off from this line of research has been discussion of the possibility that T cell receptors may have a restricted repertoire of specificities; that, for example, they can only react with foreign antigens if they are associated with other antigens which are part of the individual's own cells. This, in turn, would mean that T cell receptor V regions must be germline encoded (Section 7.2); if they were generated by random somatic variation, no such limitation to the possible range of specificities would be expected. These possibilities cannot be entirely ruled out. However, T cells must obviously learn self-tolerance, (Chapter 8) and the degree of discrimination between antigens which they must possess is established by the need to distinguish self from not self (Chapter 1), just as it is in B cells. Arguments for somatic generation of diversity would also appear to apply with equal force to T cells. It seems probable that their receptor system will turn out to obey much the same rules as for B cells.

9.5 SUMMARY

When circulating stem cells settle in the thymus they are induced to proliferate and differentiate into T lymphocytes. Immunocompetent T cells may be distinguished from B in many ways, most usefully by their different surface antigens. T cells appear to have specific surface receptors which bind antigens, and although there has been a great deal of controversy about the nature of these molecules, it now appears that they have V regions resembling those of B cell Ig, attached perhaps to a different constant region. T cells, like B, show specific memory and tolerance. Their functions may be divided into two main groups: regulation of (probably all) immune responses, and "cell-mediated immunity," reactions with antigen where B cells are not involved. These latter kinds of reactivity are transferable from one individual to another only by T cells, not by serum, and are responsible for states of delayed-type hypersensitivity in which exposure to antigen will cause release of nonspecific pharmacologically active substances from previously sensitized T cells. Certain "cytotoxic" T cells also kill foreign cells by direct contact.

FURTHER READING

9.1   Binz, H. and Wigzell, H. (1975). Shared idiotypic determinants on B and T lymphocytes reactive against the same antigenic determinants. *J. Exp. Med.* **142**, 197.

9.2   Blanden, R. V. and Gardner, I. D. (1976). The cell-mediated immune response to ectromelia virus infection. *Cell Immunol.* **22**, 271.

9.3   Cantor, H. and Weissman, I. (1976). Development and function of subpopulations of thymocytes and T lymphocytes. *Prog. Allergy* **20**, 1.

9.4   Origins of lymphocyte diversity. (1976). *Cold Spring Harbor Symp. Quant. Biol.* **41.** This volume discusses recent work on many aspects of immunology, and is a particularly good starting point for further reading on the subjects covered in Sections 9.2.1 and 9.4.5.

9.5 Cunningham, A. J. and Lafferty, K. J. (1977). A simple, conservative explanation of the H-2 restriction of interactions between lymphocytes. *Scand. J. Immunol.* **6**, 1.

9.6 Davies, A. J. S. and Carter, R. L. (eds.). (1973). Thymus dependency. *Contemp. Top. Immunobiol.* **2.** A series of articles by different authors on the thymus, T lymphocytes and thymic "hormone."

9.7 Granger, G. A., Daynes, R. A., Runge, P. E., Prieur, A-M., and Jeffes, E. W. B. (1975). Lymphocyte effector molecules and cell-mediated immune reactions. *Contemp. Top. Mol. Immunol.* **4**, 205.

9.8 Lance, E. M., Medawar, P. B., and Taub, R. N. (1973). Antilymphocyte serum. *Adv. Immunol.* **17**, 1. A comprehensive review.

9.9 Medawar, P. B. and Simpson, E. (1975). Thymus-dependent lymphocytes. *Nature (London)* **258**, 106. A classification of T cell subsets.

9.10 Miller, J. F. A. P. (1967). The thymus: yesterday, today and tomorrow. *Lancet* **ii**, 1299.

9.11 Moller, G. (ed.). (1973). Effector cells in cell-mediated immunity. *Transplant. Rev.* **17.** A collection of papers on T cell cytotoxicity.

9.12 Moller, G. (ed.). (1976). Specificity of effector T lymphocytes. *Transplant. Rev.* **29.** A collection of recent reviews, particularly on the areas covered by Sections 9.4.4 and 9.4.5.

9.13 Shortman, K., von Boehmer, H., Lipp. J., and Hopper, K. (1975). Subpopulations of T lymphocytes. *Transplant. Rev.* **25**, 163. Discusses the development of thymus lymphocytes. This volume contains a number of papers on the separation of subpopulations of T and B lymphocytes.

QUESTIONS

9.1 Mice which have been thymectomized, heavily irradiated, and then injected with bone marrow cells (to restore hemopoietic function) will survive, but now reject tissue grafts from other strains of mice very weakly or not at all. Why? Nude mice also do not reject foreign grafts. Would the implantation of a thymus allow them to develop graft rejecting powers?

9.2 If an immune response involves the production of antibodies with idiotypes that are new to the animal, and if these idiotypes, therefore, act in turn as "antigens" which provoke anti-idiotype production, what effects might the anti-idiotype antibodies have on the immune response?

9.3 Consider a compound antigen, XY, such that either X or Y alone are immunogenic. Now an animal previously made tolerant to X may produce antibody to X if stimulated with XY, the usual explanation being, as we have seen, that B cells with anti-X specificity were intact and T cells missing, but substituted for by anti-Y T cells, in this case. If, however, injection of XY *failed* to induce anti-X antibody in X-tolerant mice what would you suspect? There are two possible answers to this question, i.e., two cellular mechanisms which could account for the result. How could they be distinguished? (*Hint:* consider the response to the Y part of the antigen.)

9.4 A mouse that has been infected with mycobacterial organisms may develop a systemic state of delayed hypersensitivity to the bacterial antigens. If such an individual is injected intravenously with killed mycobacteria, together with a sufficient dose of pathogenic *Listeria* organisms to kill a normal animal, it will be resistant to the *Listeria* infection. Why?

10

Transplantation Immunology

10.1 GRAFT REJECTION

In an outbred population like the human species, every individual is genetically unique (apart from identical twins): each has a different pattern of genes, coding for different proteins. Therefore, it is not surprising that an organ or tissue is often rejected when grafted from one person to another. The new host ''sees'' most transferred material as antigenically foreign.

There are some exceptions. The body will normally accept nonliving tissues like bone and arterial wall. Similarly, transplants of nonvascularized material, like cornea, are often accepted by unrelated individuals. This implies that the free-floating cells of blood and lymph have to enter a tissue to recognize it as foreign. Second, a graft will ''take'' if it comes from another part of the *same* individual (as in skin transplantation from healthy to damaged areas on a burnt patient), or if donor and recipient are genetically identical. This shows that the mechanics of transplantation are no barrier to success. With modern surgical techniques, transplantation of kidneys and even heart is perfectly feasible: approximately 50% of transplanted kidneys from unrelated human donors are still functioning after 2 years. However, retention of these foreign grafts depends entirely on suppressing the recipient's immune reactions with drugs and other treatments (Section 10.11); we have not yet learned to control the specific immunological rejection. Evidently this is a fundamental problem in immunology. It involves a basic property of the immune system, the acquired ability to tolerate one's own tissues while reacting against foreign material. Since we are concerned mainly with the principles of the subject, we will concentrate here on integrating the phenomenology of transplantation with the rest of immunological theory.

TABLE 10.1
Terms Used in Transplantation Immunology

Prefix	Meaning	Nouns (+ synonyms)	Adjectives (+ synonyms)	Immunogenetic relationship
Auto-	Self	Autograft	Autogeneic (autochthonous) (autologous)	Self to self
Iso-	Same	Isograft	Isogeneic (syngeneic)	Different individuals but genetically identical
Allo-[a]	Other	Allograft (homograft)	Allogeneic	Same species but genetically different
Xeno-	Foreign	Xenograft (heterograft)	Xenogeneic (heterologous)	Different species

[a] Compare "allotype" (Chapter 3) which means different genetic variants of corresponding proteins from genetically different members of the same species. "Alloantigen" is also seen, as a term for antigenic variants of a protein within a species.

10.2 TERMINOLOGY

The jargon of transplantation can be confusing at first. Table 10.1 summarizes the most common terms. Different prefixes are used to denote differing degrees of genetic relationship between donor and host. *Auto* ("self") means that the same individual acts as both donor and recipient, as in "autograft." *Iso* (lit. "same"), or *syn* (lit. "together") both refer to different individuals which are genetically identical; grafts between "syngeneic" or "isogeneic" individuals are not rejected. *Allo* (lit. "other") means animals of the same species but genetically different: all humans (except identical twins) are "allogeneic" in relation to one another, and such grafts are "allografts" (or "homografts", older term). *Xeno* (foreign) means different species. Xenografts are rarely attempted; they would be physiologically as well as immunologically incompatible with the host in most cases.

10.3 EVIDENCE THAT GRAFT REJECTION IS AN IMMUNOLOGICAL PROCESS

The rejection of allografts is a process which displays the same features as other kinds of immune response.

10.3.1 Adaptivity

In mice, a skin graft becomes vascularized within a few days. However, if it is from a foreign strain (see Section 10.4), the circulation soon ceases, infiltration of mononuclear cells occurs (Section 10.5), necrosis begins, and the skin is sloughed off after about 9 days. A second graft from the same donor strain is typically rejected faster than the first, and may be destroyed within 3 or 4 days (Fig. 10.1). In other words, primary and secondary allograft rejection responses differ qualitatively, as do primary and secondary antibody responses.

10.3.2 Specificity

The accelerated ''second-set'' reaction is specific, like all other forms of immunological memory. A subsequent graft from a third unrelated individual will still be rejected slowly, in a ''primary'' manner.

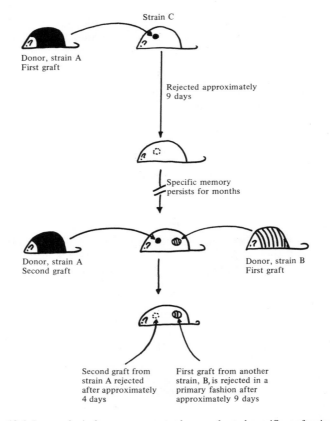

Fig. 10.1 Immunological memory expressed as accelerated specific graft rejection.

10.3.3 Diversity

Any individual can react specifically against the tissues of a great many others, although the range of antigens involved in transplantation is not unlimited, as we will see in Section 10.4.

10.3.4 Response to the Unexpected

The "transplantation" antigens (Section 10.4) of a species are constantly evolving. Mutant forms appear and spread throughout the population. The receptor (immune) system is, however, able to react against such new and "unexpected" antigens, a property which we have seen to be characteristic of the immune apparatus.

10.3.5 Tolerance

Tolerance of foreign tissues can be acquired, particularly if these tissues are present continuously from an early age (further discussed in Section 10.7).

10.3.6 Lymphocytes

The power to reject grafts in a rapid, secondary manner is transferable from an immune to a normal animal by injection of lymphocytes, reinforcing the conclusion that the phenomena are basically immunological. Similarly, nude or neonatally thymectomized mice (Section 9.3), which lack T cells, do not reject allografts. If, however, they are injected with T cells of the same kind as the host (and therefore able to attack the grafted tissue), they will reject the graft.

10.4 TRANSPLANTATION ANTIGENS

10.4.1 Genetics

This is an immensely complicated area, whose finer points can be pursued in textbooks of immunogenetics (Refs. 3.9, 3.11, and 10.5). A simplified account is given here.

Most of our knowledge comes from breeding studies with mice. If animals are mated brother to sister for many generations they become almost genetically identical, and will accept tissue grafts between one another. This inbreeding produces *homozygosity*. If the gamete from the mother has gene *A* at a particular locus, and the father's gamete also has *A* at the same locus, then the offspring will be AA, and will similarly have different pairs of identical genes at other loci. An AA animal mated with one from another strain which is BB at the same locus will yield AB progeny in the F1 generation (Fig. 10.2). As would be expected,

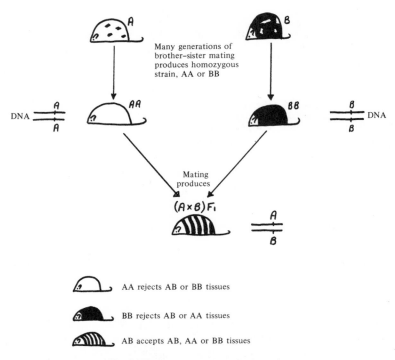

Many generations of
brother–sister mating
produces homozygous
strain, AA or BB

DNA

Mating
produces

(A×B)F₁

AA rejects AB or BB tissues

BB rejects AB or AA tissues

AB accepts AB, AA or BB tissues

Fig. 10.2 Mouse transplantation genetics.

AA accepts AA skin but rejects BB or AB. AB, however, accepts tissues from both parents, since it sees nothing foreign in either (we will qualify this statement in Section 10.7).

Breeding experiments with mice and other species show that transplantation (or *histocompatibility*) antigens are under genetic control, are inherited in Mendelian fashion, and are codominant (both alleles expressed equally). It has been established, by transferring tissues between strains and observing their rejection, or from the formation of antibody against the transplants, that the antigens involved in tissue rejection are coded for at a number of separate loci on the DNA. In mice there are at least thirteen autosomal loci, and two on the sex chromosomes. However, one group of genes codes for antigens to which the transplantation response is overwhelmingly strongest: this region is called the *major histocompatibility complex* (MHC). All mammalian species so far studied have such a dominant locus. In mice it is called the H-2 region, and is found on chromosome 17. In man it is called the HL-A region. The MHC is a stretch of DNA containing perhaps 500 adjacent genes, some of which code for histocompatibility antigens, while others play some role in the control of immune re-

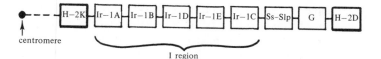

Fig. 10.3 Map of the major histocompatibility complex of the mouse. The squares represent genes or groups of genes recognized as separate from one another through the existence of mice in which recombination has taken place *within* the complex. For Chapter 10, the *H-2K* and *H-2D* genes are chiefly important: they code for all known H-2 antigens. The I region (Section 11.3.1) contains genes controlling immune responses to certain antigens, and coding also for I antigens on lymphocytes and on factors released by T cells. New subloci within this region are being recognized periodically, and the diagram represents the views of late 1976. Ss, Slp is an allotypic serum protein variant, not relevant to transplantation but serving as a useful marker in construction of the map. G is a locus coding for antigens of minor importance on red cells and lymphocytes.

sponses (the Ir genes, discussed in Section 11.3). Mice which have different H-2 regions are likely to differ so strongly in their tissue antigens that grafts are very rapidly rejected. Mice with the same H-2 genetic background which differ at other histocompatibility loci usually tolerate one another's grafts for a longer time. Figure 10.3 shows a current genetic map of the mouse MHC.

The genes responsible for histocompatibility antigens are very *polymorphic,* that is, many different alternative forms or alleles exist in a population. This polymorphism, together with the large number of separate loci which exist, means that any two unrelated animals within a species will rarely have exactly the same array of transplantation antigens. Some possible reasons for this polymorphism are discussed in Section 8.3.2 and Chapter 14.

A distinction has recently been drawn (by Bach) between two kinds of histocompatibility loci within the MHC: the first code for "serologically defined" (SD) antigens, i.e., antigens which elicit antibody formation when cells from one strain of animal are injected into another; the second code for "lymphocyte-defined" (LD) antigens, which do not stimulate antibody formation, but can be detected because lymphocytes from strains of mice differing only at LD loci will react against one another when cultured together *in vitro* (Section 10.8).

10.4.2 Nature of the Transplantation Antigens

It has been known for some years that the transplantation antigens of the major locus can be resolved into two closely linked series, called "K" and "D" in the mouse (Fig. 10.3). A similar paired arrangement is found in other species, suggesting ancestral duplication of an original single gene. These loci code for glycoproteins of about 45,000 molecular weight which are found principally on cell sufaces, as might be expected of antigens important in graft rejection. They occur on most tissues, but are particularly dense on lymphoid cells (which carry about 5×10^5 such molecules per cell). The 45,000 MW "heavy" chains are associated noncovalently on the cell surface with a 12,000 MW "light" chain molecule called β_2-microglobulin. Tetrameric forms (H_2L_2) have been described by some workers, but have been dismissed as artifacts by others.

Very recently, sequencing of mouse H-2 (and human HLA) histocompatibility antigens has begun, using isotopically labeled material purified from cell surfaces after combination with anti H-2 sera. Partial N-terminal sequences of the H chain are now available for several allelic forms (Ref. 10.5). The main conclusions so far are as follows:

1. The great serological variability of H-2 antigens is reflected in extensive sequence variation of the H chains between individuals (the microglobulin is not polymorphic within a species, and in fact is highly conserved between species).

2. K and D molecules (that is the products of the two linked alleles) are homologous, i.e., have some amino acids in common at corresponding positions, but there are no sequence patterns so far discovered which distinguish K molecules as a class from D as a class.

3. The H-2 heavy chains show no sequence homology with Ig (β_2-microglobulin does show some homology with an Ig domain, and very recently, a homology has been discovered between Ig and HL-A proteins in humans).

The particular combination of H-2 antigens at K and D loci on chromosome 17 in any one gamete constitute an H-2 "haplotype." Inbred mice are homozygous at these, as at other loci, while outbred mice have a phenotype that includes the products of four different loci, all of which are usually different in each diploid cell. The antigens coded for by H-2 region genes can be defined serologically; each glycoprotein, depending on its primary structure, induces antibodies of various specificities. Different K or D gene products sometimes share some antigenic specificities. Those antigenic specificities which are found in more than one inbred strain of mice are called *public*, while those unique to a strain are termed *private* specificities.

10.4.3 Blood Groups

While the MHC and other histocompatibility loci are mainly responsible for the acceptance or rejection of foreign organ, tissue, or lymphocyte grafts, a number of quite separate loci govern the reactions which may occur against antigens present on the surface of transfused erythrocytes. These antigens are mucopolysaccharides, their specificity being conferred by differences at the ends of the carbohydrate chains. The first human blood group polymorphism was defined by Landsteiner in 1900. This is the ABO system. As is well known, humans fall into four groups depending on whether their erythrocytes express one or both of the dominant antigens A and B, or the recessive antigen, O (Table

TABLE 10.2
Human ABO Blood Groups

Group	Erythrocyte antigens	Serum antibodies
O	–	Anti-A and anti-B
A	A	Anti-B
B	B	Anti-A
A B	A and B	–

10.2). Individuals lacking A or B normally possess IgM antibodies against the missing antigen, these antibodies being probably acquired by contact with cross-reacting material in food, dust, and gut flora. Group A blood transferred into a group O or B recipient will be lysed by antibody in the recipient's serum; thus serological typing to match donor and recipient must precede transfusion.

A number of other blood group systems are now known (for a more detailed discussion see Ref. 1.6). The Rh or rhesus system comprises several associated pairs of allelic antigens, although individuals lacking a particular antigen do not normally have antibodies against it. One of these antigens (D) is important in causing hemolytic disease of human babies. If a D^- mother gives birth to a D^+ infant, some of the fetal erythrocytes may enter the mother's circulation via placental bleeds at birth. The woman then develops anti-D IgG antibodies which can cross the placenta and destroy the erythrocytes of a subsequent D^+ fetus. D^- women with D^+ husbands may be given anti-D IgG antibody prophylactically, after the birth of the first child, to remove any fetal erythrocytes and prevent sensitization.

10.5 REJECTION MECHANISMS

As in other types of immune reactions, we can distinguish "afferent" and "efferent" phases in allograft rejection. In the afferent phase, the animal becomes sensitized; in the efferent phase, effector lymphocytes destroy the graft. The afferent phase requires that graft antigens reach the organized lymphatic tissue of the host. There, specific T lymphocytes become triggered to transform into blasts, and to divide, generating sensitized effector T cells and recirculating memory small lymphocytes (Section 9.3). Grafts in certain sites which have no lymphatic drainage ("privileged" sites) may not be rejected. Such sites include the meninges of the brain, the anterior chamber of the eye, the cheek pouch of hamsters, and, experimentally, pedicles of skin from which lymphatic drainage has been severed.

Lymphocytes, rather than antibody, seem to be the main effector agents in rejecting skin or organ grafts. This follows from the fact that adoptive immunity to an allograft can be transferred to a normal animal by lymphoid cells from a syngeneic individual immune to the same kind of graft. Similarly, tolerance may be terminated by transfer of sensitized lymphoid cells. Transfer of serum antibody alone usually has little effect on an organ graft (although antibody can cause certain hyperacute rejection processes in humans, e.g., rejection of transplanted kidneys).

That T lymphocytes rather than B cells or macrophages are responsible can be demonstrated in several ways. Treating the sensitized population before transfer with anti-θ serum (Section 9.13) will often prevent adoptive immunity. "Nude" mice (Section 9.1.3) which have no thymus, and neonatally thymectomized mice, do not reject grafts. Children with certain thymic deficiencies but with normal B cells also tolerate allografts longer than normal individuals. Conversely, bursectomized chickens (Section 5.2.5), which have T cells but no B, reject grafts normally.

However, while sensitized T cells, mainly of the cytotoxic variety (Section 9.4.4), seem to be an essential first weapon, the actual cellular events occurring in a graft which is undergoing rejection are exceedingly complex. Lymphocytes of various sizes, and many monocytes, infiltrate the tissue. There is selective retention of cells bearing receptors directed against graft antigens, as has recently been shown using the Binz–Wigzell anti-idiotype sera (Section 9.2.1). By no means are all of these T cells; many are non-T lymphocytes and monocytes or macrophages which have IgG antibody attached to their surfaces via their Fc receptors. There is also some evidence for a molecule, produced by T cells, and bearing the sinister name of SMAF (specific macrophage arming factor), which was thought to attach to macrophages and "arm" them for specific immune reactions. Cells with specific cytotoxic activity *in vitro* can be extracted from grafts, and from lymph nodes draining the site of a graft.

We should mention here a phenomenon which was discovered in connection with tumor transplantation, and which will be discussed further in Section 14.3.4. Antibody against some graft antigens, far from causing rejection, may protect or *enhance* survival of the graft. It probably does this by blocking access to cytotoxic T cells. Complexes of graft antigens with serum antibody may be more effective enhancing agents than antibody alone, although the presence of such complexes carries its own dangers; for example, a grafted kidney may fail through blockage of small blood vessels by complexes.

10.6 GRAFT VERSUS HOST REACTIONS

If immunocompetent cells are injected into a genetically (and hence antigenically) foreign host, these grafted cells may attempt "to reject the host." Transfer of allogeneic cells, e.g., AA to a BB mouse gives only a transient reaction, since the host can reject the donor cells. Injection of AA or BB cells into an AB F1 hybrid may cause a severe reaction with runting and death if the donor and recipient differ at the *H-2* locus, since the AA cells will react against the B antigens of the recipient. Here the host is genetically incompetent to react against antigens in the donor cells. Similarly, a nude, neonatally thymectomized, or very young mouse may serve as the defenseless target of attack by adult allogeneic lymphocytes. Injection of (necessarily allogeneic) bone marrow to humans can also lead to this kind of reaction.

The graft versus host response shows many of the same features as graft rejection. A similar genetic difference is required; T lymphocytes can again be shown to be the initiator cells; cells from donors tolerant of say, "A" strain allogeneic tissues, do not produce a graft versus host reaction when injected into A strain recipients.

10.7 TRANSPLANTATION TOLERANCE

As mentioned earlier, Medawar and his colleagues found that an "A" strain mouse would become tolerant of tissue from a "B" strain animal if A was injected at birth with hemopoietic tissue (e.g., bone marrow) from a B-type animal (Fig. 10.4). When the A mouse reached adulthood it would not reject B grafts. Transferring normal lymphocytes from a normal nontolerant A mouse would, however, often cause rejection of a previously tolerated graft. Lymphocytes from an A animal presensitized against B tissues by immunization in adulthood were even more effective in breaking the tolerant state. [In practice, tolerant mice for experiments of this kind were usually prepared by injecting F1 (A × B) cells into a parental (AA or BB) recipient to avoid any reaction by the grafted cells against the host (Section 10.6).]

These experiments show that the immune system can acquire tolerance to foreign tissues, as it can to other antigens, provided they are present continuously from an early age. Self-tolerance is probably acquired in the same way: an individual could react against himself, but learns not to (Section 8.2). The Medawar experiment, mentioned above, is in many respects the converse of that of Triplett (Section 6.8) who *removed* a self-component and showed that tolerance of it was lost. Permanent tolerance of the foreign transplantation antigen seems to require the establishing of a "chimeric" state, where donor lymphoid cells persist in a stable mixture with similar cells of recipient type.

10.7.1 Mechanisms

The main debate about transplantation tolerance, as with tolerance to nonliving antigens, centers around whether the specific cells reactive against the foreign

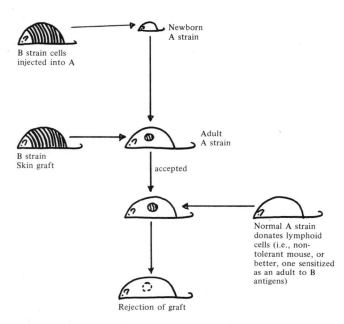

Fig. 10.4 Breaking homograft tolerance by transfer of cells from an animal not tolerant of the graft.

tissue are deleted or merely suppressed (Section 6.9.2). Injection of large numbers of lymphoid or hemopoietic cells into a newborn recipient favors a state of "complete" tolerance, subsequent donor-type grafts being indefinitely retained. Mechanistically, such tolerant animals behave as if they lacked specific anti-graft-reactive cells: their cells fail to suppress reactions by syngeneic lymphocytes from nontolerant individuals against antigens of the donor strain. By contrast, injecting a smaller number of foreign cells into older recipients induces, at best, "partial" tolerance, specific rejection of grafts being delayed but not prevented. There is some evidence for at least three kinds of suppressor mechanisms in states of this latter type:

1. Blocking substances in serum, which specifically prevent host cells reacting against the graft, and probably consist of antigen, antibody or complexes as discussed in Section 10.5.

2. Anti-idiotype antibody: we have seen (Section 9.3.2) that F1 cells may make anti-(parent-anti-F1) anti-idiotype antibody, which could conceivably prevent a parental strain host from rejecting an F1 graft. There are reports that "preimmunizing" F1 animals (A × B) with P (parental) strain (AA) lymphocytes may increase their subsequent resistance to attack by a second inoculum of the same kind of P cells.

3. Suppressor T cells have been described in several experimental systems where unresponsiveness to histocompatibility antigens was induced in adult animals.

We will discuss suppressive versus deletion tolerance in the next chapter. The situation is even more complex in transplantation tolerance than in tolerance to simple antigens, since in the former case there are living cells of both donor and host origin able to contribute to the final balanced (or unbalanced) state. Those wishing to explore this topic further should consult Refs. 10.1 and 10.4. It is sufficient here to say that there is a steady swing away from the older idea that ''true'' tolerance requires deletion of specifically reactive cells, and toward the view that it is achieved by active regulatory mechanisms.

10.7.2 Toleration of the Fetus

An interesting natural example of tolerance of a homograft is the maternal–fetal relationship. In any outbred population, the fetus will have some paternal antigens which are foreign to the mother, and in many species, the mother's circulating lymphocytes come into contact with the fetal trophoblast. It is not known why this contact is tolerated. A pregnancy is not affected by prior sensitization of the mother against paternal antigens, suggesting that there is no immunological attack against the fetus. Possibly the arrangement or amount of histocompatibility antigens on the trophoblast is such that cytotoxic lymphocytes cannot react effectively against this tissue. In some species the trophoblast seems to be protected by a sialic acid-rich mucopolysaccharide layer. We can discount the intriguing suggestions that birth is an immunological rejection, since inbred animals are born in the same way as offspring which are genetically different from their mothers.

10.8 MIXED LYMPHOCYTE REACTION

When two populations of lymphocytes, allogeneic to one another, are cultured together *in vitro,* vigorous proliferation may occur in both. This kind of reaction is thought to be caused by immunocompetent cells of one strain reacting against antigens on the cells of the other strain, and vice versa. The reaction can be made to go only ''one way,'' i.e., so that cells in only one of the two populations proliferates, either by treating one of the allogeneic partners in such a way as to inhibit its division (e.g., by prior X-irradiation), or by using combinations of parental (AA) and F1 (AB) cells, in which case it might be expected that the F1 cells could not find any foreign antigens on the parental strain cells to react against. Under some circumstances, specific cytotoxic T cells can be generated in mixed lymphocyte cultures.

10.9 ANOMALOUS FEATURES OF ALLOGENEIC
REACTIONS

We can group together as "allogeneic reactions" all those with an apparently immunological basis which occur between genetically different cells of the same species. Graft versus host and mixed lymphocyte culture reactions are studied as model systems to help understand the more complex events of graft rejection. They involve T lymphocytes, are specific, and occur only where there is some antigenic difference between partners, as we have seen. The conventional explanation would be that they represent the immune reactions of immunocompetent cells against foreign transplantation antigens. However, both graft versus host and mixed lymphocyte reactions have some anomalous properties.

1. Allogeneic combinations usually give much stronger reactions than xenogeneic ones (between species), in spite of the fact that much greater antigenic differences exist between species than between any two members of the same species. This has led to the suggestion, which is important for immunological theory (Sections 8.3.2 and 14.4), that *alloantigens* have some particular significance within a species (see below).

2. Cultured lymphocytes respond vigorously only to living, metabolically active, allogeneic lymphocytes. They do not usually proliferate if exposed to extracted alloantigens, or to dead lymphocytes, or to most kinds of allogeneic cells which are not lymphocytes (e.g., fibroblasts), that is, *stimulation* must be done by a viable lymphoid cell (or by a closely related cell type, e.g., it seems that macrophages may stimulate). This is obviously different from antibody reactions where soluble antigens provoke responses.

3. The cells *responding* (i.e., proliferating) in a mixed lymphocyte culture are usually lymphocytes which are "genetically capable" of reacting to antigens of the other population, e.g., P (parental strain) lymphocytes respond to F1. However, there are cases where immunogenetic principles seem to be contravened. In mixtures of P and F1 spleen cells, for example, both types proliferate. When parental strain adult lymphocytes are injected into F1 embryos (chickens) or newborn animals (mice) much of the damaging proliferation is done by host (F1) cells.

4. Where graft versus host or mixed lymphocyte reactions are occurring across a very strong histocompatibility antigen difference (e.g., between partners differing at *H-2* in the mouse), it is usually difficult to increase the speed or vigor of the reaction by preimmunization.

5. The most important anomaly is the fact that an extremely high proportion of lymphocytes will react against other allogeneic lymphocytes. Several estimates of this proportion have been made.

(*i*) Simonsen found that less than 100 adult lymphocytes were able to cause a graft versus host reaction when injected into baby allogeneic mice. This implies that more than 1% of lymphocytes can react to a particular set of alloantigens.

(*ii*) Wilson demonstrated that, in mixed lymphocyte cultures, 1–2% of cells are provoked into division by the presence of allogeneic lymphocytes.

(*iii*) Ford injected radiolabeled thoracic duct lymphocytes into allogeneic rats and estimated that about 12% of these were specifically trapped in host lymphoid tissues because of their reactivity against host alloantigens.

(*iv*) Wigzell, using anti-idiotype serum (Section 9.2.1), calculates that about 5% of mouse T lymphocytes have an idiotype characteristic of a particular alloantibody specificity.

10.10 POSSIBLE EXPLANATIONS FOR THE ANOMALIES IN ALLOGENEIC REACTIONS

The paradoxical features of allogeneic reactions, and, in particular, the high proportion of lymphocytes apparently reactive to alloantigens, are obviously very important to immunological theory. They seem to challenge the basic concept of the immune system as a population of diverse, specific lymphocytes. If, for example, 5% of cells interact with one small group of alloantigens, and there are many allogeneic types within a species, it would seem that each lymphocyte must recognize many different antigens. Three main kinds of explanation have been offered to encompass the unexpected features of allogeneic reactions (Fig. 10.5).

1. That there are an unusually large number of cells with receptors for alloantigens, perhaps one thousand times more than against corresponding antigens from different species. This would make alloantigens particularly "strong." How such an unbalanced repertoire of immunocompetent cells might have arisen is discussed in Chapter 14 (immune surveillance hypothesis).

This idea is firmly entrenched in the literature. Against it is the observation that alloantigens do *not* stimulate a high proportion of cells when removed from lymphocyte surfaces and presented in purified form. Also it does not easily account for cases where F1 cells respond to parental type stimulators.

2. That an entirely separate nonimmunological recognition system is involved. This radical assumption ignores the fact that allogeneic reactions *do* show many conventional immune properties notably tolerance, and mediation by lymphocytes. Any plausible alternative scheme would have to say how such immunological elements could be incorporated.

3. Figure 10.5 shows a recent interpretation of allogeneic reactions (by Dr. K. J. Lafferty and the author) which attempts to explain their peculiar features in terms of known immunological mechanisms (Refs. 10.2, 10.8). The reader should be warned that this is a personal view, and not by any means widely accepted. It is presented here because it demonstrates, hopefully in a heuristic

Basic phenomenon: 1% or more of A strain cells proliferate when
                         brought into contact with allogeneic D cells

Possible explanations:

(1) 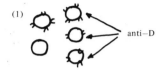 anti—D   Many more cells with anti—D receptors
                                   than with receptors to other antigens

(2) 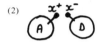   Another, nonimmunological recognition
                                   system is operating, e.g., between x^+
                                   and x^- units, displayed by A and B
                                   strain cells respectively; much less
                                   diversity

(3)   A mixed lymphocyte reaction is simply a normal inductive-
           type reaction between lymphocytes in which the antigens
           involved are cell-surface components

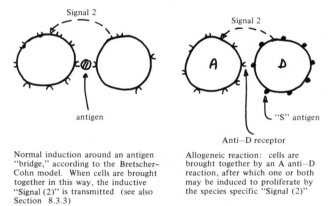

Normal induction around an antigen   Allogeneic reaction: cells are
"bridge," according to the Bretscher-   brought together by an A anti—D
Cohn model. When cells are brought   reaction, after which one or both
together in this way, the inductive   may be induced to proliferate by
"Signal (2)" is transmitted (see also   the species specific "Signal (2)"
Section 8.3.3)

Fig. 10.5 Possible explanations for some of the anomalous features of allogeneic reactions.

way, many of the principles of immunology which we have already encountered.
It is assumed that vertebrate lymphocytes stimulate one another when brought
close together in a certain way. This stimulatory mechanism has evolved for the
purpose of immune induction, and we have seen (Chapter 5) that there is ample
evidence for some such cell–cell interaction in immune responses. In normal

induction, this contact of cells occurs around an antigen bridge; allogeneic reactions may simply be an abnormal form of this process (Fig. 10.5). The antigens are cell surface components; one of the interacting pair must have antibody receptors for antigens on the other, but it does not matter which; thus F1 cells which lack receptors for P, can "respond," i.e., proliferate after close contact with a P-strain cell which binds to antigens on the F1. The induction signal is species-specific, and is the same "signal 2" (Bretscher and Cohn, Section 8.3.3) as has been postulated for normal induction. The stimulator cell must be metabolically active in order to transmit this signal. It is obvious, based on this view, why isolated alloantigens are not stimulatory.

The high proportion of cells reacting is a result of two things. First, the large number of molecules of alloantigens on a cell surface, which allows many individual receptors to bind to antigen, creating a firm overall bond, even when the affinity of each single reaction is low (more than 1% of cells are known to bind other randomly selected proteins when they are displayed on a surface in this way). We have already encountered this idea, that binding of immunocompetent cells to polymeric antigens is highly "degenerate," i.e., not very specific (Sections 2.3.3 and 5.5.2), and we will discuss it further at the beginning of the next chapter. Second, the fact that any binding between allogeneic lymphoid cells, however weak, results in induction, since transmission of "signal 2" automatically follows this kind of contact.

Whatever the detailed mechanism of allogeneic reactions it is clear that lymphocytes from genetically different members of the same species stimulate one another strongly. This has important implications for graft rejection. The lymphocytes in the *donor* tissue may contribute to its rejection (see Section 10.11.1).

10.11 PREVENTING GRAFT REJECTION

There is no foolproof and general procedure yet known to prevent allograft rejection between histoincompatible recipients. However, there are several ways of lessening rejection; they will be discussed briefly in the sections that follow.

10.11.1 Preventing Stimulation by the Graft

If donor and recipient are the same, no immune rejection occurs. Therefore, the closer one can get to this relationship the better. Human tissues are often selected on the basis of matching procedures similar to those used in blood grouping, e.g., lymphocytes from the donor and recipient may be tested against a battery of alloantisera to select that donor most similar to the intended recipient.

For organ grafts there is a promising new approach to minimizing the strength of rejection reactions which has been pioneered by Summerlin, Lafferty and

TABLE 10.3
Preventing Rejection of Thyroid Allografts by Organ Culture *In Vitro* Prior to Transplantation[a]

Period of culture (days)	Strain of recipient mouse	Initial number of grafts transplanted	Number of recipients with a surviving graft after	
			20 days	60 days
0	BALB/c	11	11	11
	CBA	8	0	0
26	BALB/c	7	7	7
	CBA	5	5	5

[a]The thyroid grafts were all from BALB/c strain of mouse donors, and were transplanted under the kidney capsules of either BALB/c (syngeneic) or CBA (allogeneic) recipients, one graft per mouse. Survival of a graft was assessed histologically and by its ability to incorporate radiolabeled iodine (from Lafferty *et al.*, Ref. 10.7).

others. It has been known for some years that the lymphocytes within a graft ("passenger leukocytes") are important in the reaction which leads to rejection, possibly because they engage in a damaging mixed lymphocyte reaction with the host's lymphocytes, and because antigen on allogeneic lymphocytes is best placed to induce cytotoxic T cells. Recent work has shown that culturing thyroid for several weeks *in vitro* before transplanting into a foreign host makes it much less liable to rejection (Ref. 10.7), probably because the graft's lymphocytes die (Table 10.3).

10.11.2 General Immunosuppression

Since lymphocytes have to divide in the process of generating effector cells, we might anticipate that preventing cell division would stop graft rejection. Thus cytotoxic drugs like azathioprine and methotrexate are used to treat human recipients of homografts. This shotgun approach has two undesirable consequences. First, all types of dividing cells are killed by the drug, which produces dangerous side effects. Second, all immune reactions, and not only the specific rejection of the graft, are suppressed, which means that the patient is more susceptible to infections. Antilymphocyte serum (Section 9.1.3), which is now quite widely used in human clinical medicine, avoids the first of these problems, but not the second.

10.11.3 Specific Immunosuppression

Quite clearly, the ideal way to prevent rejection of a graft is to suppress that particular immune reaction and not any other. Acquiring the knowledge necessary for this kind of clinical manipulation is a major aim of basic immunology. An obvious approach would be make the prospective recipient tolerant of a graft with soluble antigens from the donor before transplanting an organ. This has been tried, but thus far without great success. Enhancing antibody or antigen–antibody complexes would also seem to have potential; the ideal would be to immunize the prospective recipient against donor tissues before grafting. However, we still do not know enough to be confident that a particular immunization regime would reliably induce enhancing antibody rather than cytotoxic cells, or that a certain serum could be guaranteed to have a protective action on a graft rather than the reverse. Given the intrinsic unpredictability of immune responses (Chapter 11), this kind of approach may never be feasible.

A third way of helping graft survival may be to immunize the host against the idiotypes of those receptors on its cells which would otherwise reject the graft. Binz and Wigzell (Section 9.2.1) have some encouraging results: rats of strain A were immunized against the idiotype of specific (A-anti-B) antibodies. These rats now tolerated B strain skin grafts longer than usual.

10.12 SUMMARY

The rejection of grafted foreign tissue is basically an immunological phenomenon. It is adaptive, specific, and mediated by lymphocytes. Tolerance of a graft can be induced in its host. The antigens principally involved are coded for at a number of loci, but particularly at one complex locus which has many alleles; it is the great diversity provided by combinations of these alleles which accounts for the fact that virtually every individual in an outbred population is antigenically unique. Certain features of the reactions between lymphocytes from different individuals of a species appear anomalous, in particular, the fact that more than 1% of all lymphocytes may react against one set of foreign alloantigens. Three possible explanations for this are discussed. The lymphocytes *within* a graft may contribute to its rejection.

FURTHER READING

10.1   Brent, L., Brooks, C. G., Medawar, P. B., and Simpson, E. (1976). Transplantation tolerance. *Brit. Med. Bull.* **32,** 101. A clear, short review. This volume contains a number of useful papers on transplantation generally.

10.2   Cunningham, A. J. (1975). Why do so many cells take part in mixed lymphocyte reactions? *Cell. Immunol.* **19,** 368. For a much longer discussion of the problem, see Ref. 10.8.

10.3   Grebe, S. C. and Streilein, J. W. (1976). Graft-versus-host reactions: a review. *Adv. Immunol.* **22,** 120.

10.4   Hayry, P. (1976). Problems and prospects in surgical immunology. *Med. Biol.* **54,** 1. A comprehensive review on transplantation.

10.5   Howard, J. C. (1976). H-2 and HLA sequences. *Nature (London)* **261,** 189.
10.6   Klein, J. (1975). "Biology of the Mouse Histocompatibility - 2 Complex." Springer-Verlag, Berlin, Heidelberg and New York.
10.7   Lafferty, K. J., Bootes, A., Killby, V. A. A., and Burch, W. (1976). "Mechanism of allograft rejection." *Aust. J. Exp. Biol. Med. Sci.* **54,** 573.
10.8   Lafferty, K. J., and Cunningham, A. J. (1975). "A new analysis of allogeneic interactions." *Aust. J. Exp. Biol. Med. Sci.* **53,** 27.

QUESTIONS

10.1   Why is it that a kidney donated by a brother or sister has a better chance of being accepted by a patient than one from a randomly selected donor? Would a kidney graft from a grandparent be equally acceptable?

10.2   A kidney from a rat of strain AA is grafted into an F1 host, AB, where it functions without being rejected. The same kidney is then transplanted back into the original donor. What might happen to it, and why?

10.3   You have three cages of mice, on which the labels have become mixed up, but you remember that one was strain "AA" and the other two hybrids of genotypes "AB" and "BC." You decide to sort them out by establishing a series of graft versus host reactions in which 10^8 lymphoid cells from mice of each strain are injected into individuals of each of the other two strains. The results obtained are shown in the table below. There are three categories of effect: −, no reaction; +, a vigorous but transient reaction; third, death of the injected mouse. Which group is which?

Cells injected from box	Hosts from box		
	1	2	3
1	−	−	+
2	Death	−	+
3	+	+	−

(*Clue:* Consider first what kind of relationship must exist between donor and recipient if the donor lymphocytes survive in the recipient long enough to kill it.)

11

Regulation of the Immune Response

The major practical aim of immunology is to understand the immune system well enough to predict the outcome of any response, and ultimately to control responses as accurately as possible. We might hope, for example, to learn how to improve immunity against microorganisms, parasites, and tumors, and to prevent such harmful reactions as autoimmune disease (Chapter 12), allergies (Chapter 12), and homograft rejection (Chapter 10). There are two, related obstacles to the realization of these laudable ambitions. First, it is becoming clear that the induction of an immune response is a very complex process which depends on many factors over and above the antigen itself. Second, it now seems that immune responses are highly regulated, and require elaborate interactions between cells at all stages. These complexities make it very difficult to predict just what antibody a given antigen will induce.

This chapter is divided into three main sections. First, the indeterminate nature of immune induction is briefly discussed. Next we examine some of the burgeoning evidence for active suppression in immunological phenomena. Finally, we will touch on control of responses at the genetic level. Because the whole subject of immune regulation is both new and rapidly evolving, it is inevitable that this chapter will be more speculative than most. We will concentrate on possible principles behind the regulatory events rather than on mechanistic details, about which opinions are likely to change very rapidly.

11.1 DEGENERACY OF IMMUNE RESPONSES

There is a legacy of what might be called "chemical determinism" in today's immunology. Around the time of Landsteiner and Heidelberger (1930's) there were great advances in knowledge of antibody and its behavior: antigen and antibody were shown to react in a simple, quantitative, chemical way. They could be thought of as combining like lock and key. This kind of "model," which works well in explaining serological reactions, has since been directly applied to the much more complex area of immune induction. Antigen was thought to be the only important factor in determining what antibodies are made, acting like a key which "turned on" only those cells into whose receptors the antigenic determinants could fit exactly. In practice, however, when the same antigen is given in the same amounts to genetically identical animals, they do not usually produce the same antibodies. Instead, each animal makes a unique mixture of many different antibodies, with varying degrees of affinity for the antigen. We may refer to this lack of reproducibility in the outcome of immune responses under apparently identical conditions as *degeneracy*.

This concept of degeneracy is not normally stressed, but must be understood if we are to grasp the essential nature of the immune response. The word was initially used (Little and Eisen and Gershon) to emphasize that any one antibody can react with a variety of different antigenic determinants. By analogy with the description of the genetic code as "degenerate" in the sense that one amino acid can be represented by any one of several codons in the DNA, we can say that the immune response is "degenerate" because one antigen induces many different antibodies, or, alternatively, because there are many ways to make an immune response to a given antigen. The term encompasses the general unpredictability and variability of responses, and the lack of any exact correspondence between antigen and antibody, and between an antigen and the antibodies it will *induce*.

Why this unpredictability? Why is the immune system different from, say, the endocrine system, where a certain inducer molecule reliably provokes the release of a particular hormone? In part, the uncertainties of immune induction reflect the complexity of the processes taking place. Table 11.1 lists some of the possible factors involved; we have encountered most of them in earlier chapters. For example, a hapten coupled to a self-component may engender tolerance, or a state of delayed hypersensitivity, while the same hapten coupled to a foreign protein will induce vigorous anti-hapten, IgG antibody formation, provided there are sufficient carrier-reactive helper T cells available. If the hapten is presented coupled to a polymeric, thymus-independent carrier, the antibody made will be largely IgM and of low affinity. Different individual animals will treat the same antigen in slightly different ways; e.g., some may have more helper cells of a particular specificity than others because of a prior infection with, say, a bacterium bearing cross-reacting antigens; each individual will have a different array of lymphocytes created by random genetic processes (at least in the opinion of many immunologists); there must be an element of chance in what lymphocytes an antigen happens to encounter in the body, particularly if little antigen is present (as is the case in many natural infections). "Chance" (which is another way of saying events whose causes we cannot exactly determine), plays an important part throughout biology, from the shuffling of the genes upward. In

Table 11.1
Factors Influencing Immune Responses

A. The antigen
   1. Amount (not a simple relationship between amount of antigen and size of response; e.g., too much may cause tolerance)
   2. Molecular size (small compounds nonimmunogenic; cell–cell cooperation not possible)
   3. Physical form (polymers usually more immunogenic; multipoint binding)
   4. Mitogenic activity (ability to stimulate cell division nonspecifically)
   5. Relationship to "self": if close, poorly immunogenic
   6. Ease of degradation (highly stable antigens tend to cause tolerance, because they persist)
   7. Chemical fine structure (the "determinant" composition)
   8. Other side effects of antigen, e.g., local inflammatory action; more cells recruited

B. The individual immunocompetent cell
   1. Affinity of its receptors
   2. Arrangement of surface receptors (e.g., clustering may promote strong binding of antigen)
   3. Fluidity of its plasma membrane
   4. Stage of its life history on meeting antigen (memory cells may be more easily induced, and newly generated cells more readily inactivated)
   5. Stage of mitotic cycle (?)

C. The population of cells meeting antigen
   1. Relative proportions of different types (e.g., T and B; whether the antigen is "presented" by macrophages?)
   2. Absolute numbers of relevant immunocompetent cells available
   3. Anatomical distribution of cells and antigen (e.g., sessile cells only meet local antigen; intradermal antigen may stimulate delayed hypersensitivity)
   4. Degree of competition between cells for antigen (small amounts favor high affinity cells; clones may "compete" with one another after induction)
   5. Amount and rapidity of suppressor reactions stimulated
   6. *Uncertainty* elements (e.g., production of variants within a clone which can then be selected)

D. The whole animal
   1. Past antigenic experience
   2. Age, species, sex, hormonal state
   3. Genetic composition (especially Ir genes)

immune induction, however, its effects are especially marked. This topic is discussed further in Ref. 2.1.

There seems also to be another important reason for the degeneracy of immune responses: lack of specificity in the initial combination between antigen and immunocompetent cells. The reader should critically appraise the following section for himself since it represents the author's personal views. It is customary, particularly in introductory textbooks, to stress that antibody molecules can be highly specific, in the sense that they may discriminate between chemically similar compounds (Section 2.3.5). This sort of observation led naturally to the idea that antigen stimulates cells with equal discrimination, a protein, for example, selecting perhaps one cell in a million from a population and inducing its clonal proliferation. However, we have seen that combination between multivalent antigens and an array of receptors on a lymphocyte surface is a much more permissive affair than monovalent hapten combining site union (Fig. 2.10). The experimental facts are that a single protein antigen, if present in high concentration, or as a matrix array on a surface, will bind to 1% or more of mouse splenic lymphocytes (Section 5.2.2); from 1 to 10% of such lymphocytes react with alloantigens (when these are displayed on a foreign lymphocyte surface, Section 10.9); recent observations show that a single particulate antigen, such as sheep erythrocytes, will provoke Ig synthesis by as many as 10% of mature B lymphocytes. Clearly, the initial stimulation of the immune system by a large dose of antigen involves a fairly large proportion of immunocompetent cells: there is vigorous proliferation, perhaps generation of lymphocytes with new, variant specificities (Section 8.3.5), and, as the amount of antigen falls, eventual selection of a tiny proportion of cells to make the high affinity and often highly specific antibody that is eventually measured. In the author's opinion, the purpose of this early activity is to *create,* by genetic variation, lymphocytes of entirely new specificities that can then be selected by antigen, although this thesis, which is defended in Ref. 8.4, is not yet accepted by most immunologists.

11.2 SUPPRESSOR REGULATION OF IMMUNE RESPONSES

Obviously one's views on the extent to which immune responses are "preprogrammed" will strongly influence one's expectations of the importance of regulation. If immune induction involves simply the precise selection of a rare lymphocyte specificity from among millions, followed by several rounds of self-limited division in that clone, then there is little need for controls. If, on the other hand, an immune reaction is a haphazard affair, the animal learning to adapt to the antigen as the response proceeds, then regulation will be seen as very important, in particular, to control any anti-self reactions that may arise. The recent evolution of ideas in this area is fascinating, and may be considered under the following three headings.

1. The original "single-hit" view: Immunological mechanisms used to seem delightfully simple until 10 or 15 years ago. Cells were induced by a single hit with antigen, whereupon they expanded into a clone of active antibody forming cells (Fig. 11.1). Antigen was removed in a simple feedback loop by excess antibody. Self-tolerance was thought to be assured by the destruction of

(1) "Purge" theory (Lederberg, Burnet)

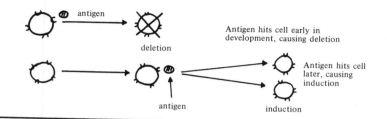

(2) Bretscher–Cohn scheme

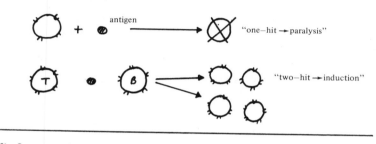

(3) Suppressor tolerance

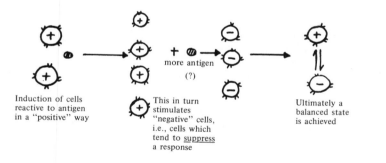

Fig. 11.1 Possible mechanisms of tolerance.

cells which met antigen before a certain (early) stage in development of the individual (Section 8.3.1). Any foreign antigen present before this critical stage would also "purge" cells reactive to it, this being the explanation offered for the early finding of Medawar and others that a neonatal injection of foreign hemopoietic cells often made a recipient animal permanently tolerant of the donor's tissues (Section 10.7). Three main lines of evidence eventually undermined this simple view: (a) the finding that tolerance could be induced in adult animals. At first it was thought only massive doses of antigen would do this, and adult tolerance was called "paralysis" in the belief that it was a different phenomenon, but later it was found that low initial doses of antigen could also decrease the specific responsiveness of adults (Section 6.7.2); (b) the discovery of cell cooperation in the induction of immune responses (Section 5.5), which showed that the induction of a cell involved more than simple contact with antigen; (c) the observation that tolerance is often maintained by active suppression (Section 6.9 and below).

2. The "one-hit tolerance, two-hit induction" view: The work on cell collaboration inspired the Bretscher–Cohn theory which we have already reviewed in Section 8.3.3. Collaboration between T and B cells was now considered necessary for induction, while tolerance was caused by inactivation of cells which met antigen alone in the absence of another collaborating cell. This could occur at any stage of the animal's life. Adult tolerance in two zones (Section 6.7.2) was elegantly accounted for since very high doses of antigen would coat all cells, and thus prevent cell–cell bridging, while very low doses would be statistically unlikely to bring cells together. Self-tolerance was established by deletion of cells reactive to self as they arose, one by one. All self-antigens were assumed to be present by the time lymphocytes acquired receptors, so that an animal would never accumulate a sufficient number of cells with anti-self reactivity to make inductive interactions probable.

Many immunologists still believe that this theory, or something similar, is adequate to account for self—not self discrimination. The main reason for questioning it has been the snowballing evidence for active suppression in tolerance states (Sections 6.9 and 10.7).

3. Active suppression: The bottom portion of Fig. 11.1 shows a different kind of view of the regulation of an immune response. Antigen first induces cells to differentiate, and this induction is probably aided by cell–cell collaboration. The increased number of specific antigen-reactive cells somehow provokes a "negative" response on the part of other cells, i.e., cells are generated which tend to "turn off" the response, and eventually a balance between the two types is maintained. There is ample evidence for such active suppression now, although just how it works is still obscure. Some possible mechanisms are discussed in Section 11.2.2.

11.2.1 Active Suppression in Immunological Tolerance

To recapitulate: opinions of the mechanisms of tolerance can be divided into two broad classes, "deletion" and "suppression." In both cases, animals do not respond to the particular antigen, but in the former it is because reactive cells are missing, while in the latter it is because specific suppressor cells have been generated. This difference is readily tested by experiment, the most commonly used test being one which we encountered in Section 6.9 and in Fig. 6.4. Deletion tolerance should be "recessive," that is, adding a tolerant population of cells to normal cells should not affect the response to antigen of the normals. Suppressor tolerance should be "dominant" (sometimes called "active" or even "infectious"): the tolerant population may suppress the response of a normal population. Table 11.2 provides an example, in which a hapten–carrier cooperation experiment was established by injecting carrier-primed and hapten-primed cells, together with the linked antigen, into irradiated recipient mice (Section 5.4.3). The response could be depressed by adding spleen cells from a mouse tolerant to the carrier protein.

Another way of demonstrating active suppression of immune responses is presented in some detail (in Fig. 11.2 and Table 11.3) because it is highly instructive. Suppressor cells reactive against antigen X may diminish a response to a second antigen Y if the two antigens are coupled together (see also Section 9.3). Apparently the responses made by B cells may be either helped or suppressed by other cells which recognize parts of the same antigen molecule.

Suppressor effects such as those outlined above have now been described in a wide variety of experimental situations involving tolerance to proteins, polysac-

TABLE 11.2
Suppression of Collaborative Anti-DNP Splenic PFC Responses by HGG-Tolerant Spleen Cells[a]

Group	HGG-tolerant spleen cells (suppressors)	HGG-primed spleen cells (helpers)	DNP-primed B cells	Anti-DNP plaque forming cells per spleen after 7 days
1	—	2×10^7	5×10^6	33,980
2	10^8	2×10^7	5×10^6	2,370
2	10^8	—	5×10^6	660
4	—	—	5×10^6	100

[a] Cells *tolerant* of HGG (human gamma-globulin, a commonly used protein antigen) were obtained from mice injected with 2.5 mg of a solution from which aggregated material had been removed by ultracentrifugation. The suppressor activity has been shown, in other experiments, to be associated with T cells.

Cells *primed* to HGG were made by injecting other mice with a smaller dose of the antigen mixed with an adjuvant.

Primed anti-DNP B cells were induced by injecting mice with DNP (dinitrophenyl hapten) coupled to a different protein, flagellin. (Cells from these mice were treated with anti-θ serum to remove T cells.)

Cells were mixed as shown above, and injected into irradiated, syngeneic, recipient animals together with DNP-HGG. IgG plaque forming cells to the DNP were counted 7 days later. (After Basten *et al.*, Ref. 11.4.)

<u>Step 1</u>   Induce tolerance to X.   Possible effects on cells include:

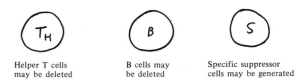

Helper T cells may be deleted	B cells may be deleted	Specific suppressor cells may be generated

<u>Step 2</u>   Challenge tolerant animals with two antigens, X and Y, either of which can induce a response when injected alone into normal animals. The two antigens are given as a simple mixture X + Y to some individuals, and coupled together, XY, to other individuals.

Nature of the tolerant state	Antibody made			
	Against X		Against Y	
	Challenge with X + Y	Challenge with XY	Challenge with X + Y	Challenge with XY
(T̶H̶) (B) Anti-X T cells deleted	−	+	+	+
(TH) (B̶) Anti-X B cells deleted	−	−	+	+
(TH) (B) (S) Anti-X Suppressors present	−	−	+	−

Fig. 11.2 Linked antigen experiment for "diagnosing" state of tolerance to an antigen, X.

charides, erythrocytes, tumors, and allogeneic tissues (reviewed in Refs. 11.2, 11.4, and 11.13). Not only is antibody formation susceptible to this sort of control, but delayed hypersensitivity reactions can also be actively suppressed. There is some evidence that such suppressor cells are generated during the course of normal immune responses; for example, treatments like irradiation or injection of antilymphocyte serum, which kill some lymphocytes, may actually increase responses if given during the early stages of a response, suggesting that lymphocytes with "negative" activity are predominant at certain times. They may be essential for regulation of all responses.

11.2.2 Possible Mechanisms of Suppression

Perhaps the most important questions here are the following: What kinds of cell cause suppression? On what other cells do they act? How do they exert their effects, in particular, what specificity do they show?

While cases of suppression by immune complexes and macrophages are known, in most instances it seems that T cells are responsible. There is recent

TABLE 11.3
An Example of the Effect of Tolerance to One Antigen on the Response to a Second Antigen Linked to the First[a]

Dose of lysozyme used to create tolerance in newborn mice (mg)	Anti-lysozyme titers ± SD		Anti-BSA titers ± SD	
	(1) Challenge with mixture	(2) Challenge with conjugate	(3) Challenge with mixture	(4) Challenge with conjugate
Control	24.0±5.0	36.0±27.0	13.0±5.0	5.0±3.0
5	0	7.9± 5.0	8.1±1.3	1.5±2.0
20	0	1.8± 1.3	11.5±6.4	0.4±0.4

[a] Mice were made tolerant to lysozyme by injection of 5 or 20 mg soon after birth. At 6 weeks of age they were challenged with either a mixture of lysozyme and BSA (bovine serum albumin), or with a covalently coupled lysozyme-BSA conjugate, using a small dose of the antigens to which mice not made tolerant would normally respond. Anti-lysozyme and anti-BSA titers are recorded as amounts of radiolabeled antigen bound by serum antibody.

Column (1) shows that the tolerant mice were unable to respond to lysozyme alone. Column (2) demonstrates that when the lysozyme was coupled to BSA, some anti-lysozyme response occurred. One interpretation of this result would be that anti-lysozyme T cells have been deleted, but that anti-BSA T cells can substitute for them and induce anti-lysozyme B cells to make antibody. The bottom result in this column would be consistent with deletion of specific B cells as well (see Fig. 11.2).

The anti-BSA titers in column (3) show that a response against BSA alone was not affected by the state of tolerance to lysozyme. However, when animals were challenged with conjugate, anti-BSA titers were depressed, implying that anti-lysozyme suppressor cells were present [column (4)]. This table should be studied after reviewing Fig. 11.2. SD=standard deviation. (Data from Scibienski *et al.*, Ref. 11.19.)

evidence that suppressor and helper T cells are different; for example, they can be separated by physical fractionation methods (Section 5.2) and have different surface markers, such as Ly antigens (Section 9.1.3). Apart from indications that T cells recently released from the thymus are precursors of suppressor T cells, little is known of their developmental history.

For suppressor cells to exert specific effects it would seem that they must, like helper cells, react with antigen via specific receptors. This reaction would be followed by the generation of some kind of "negative" signal, inhibiting associated cells from being induced by the antigen. Some evidence exists for antigen-specific suppressor signals (Section 11.3.4). There is, however, a second possibility. Suppressor cells may act against the *idiotype* (Section 9.2.1) of a cell which recognizes antigen, that is, if B or T cells recognize antigen X via their surface receptors, they may be prevented from reacting to X by a suppressor cell with specificity anti- (anti-X).

There are some experimental examples of suppression of specific immune responses by such anti-idiotype antibody. The hapten phosphorylcholine stimulates antibodies which are mainly of one particular idiotype (Section 11.2.4).

Antibody against the idiotype, if administered to unimmunized mice, will prevent their making the idiotype after immunization with phosphorylcholine. Rats of strain L immunized with antigens from another strain, BN, first make anti-BN, then anti-anti-BN, which causes disappearance of the original antibody. These and other results have prompted Jerne and Lindenmann to devise a beautiful theoretical scheme of immune regulation in which all immunocompetent cells form part of a network, each being controlled by other cells with specific activity against the idiotype of its receptors, and these in turn being controlled by anti-anti-idiotype cells, etc. The array would not be infinite, but would link like a net, e.g., the fourth cell in a line of "anti-antis" might itself have antibody activity for another foreign antigen. Introducing an antigen into the system would stimulate not only the directly complementary cells, but also, indirectly, all nearby controlling elements. A "ripple" would thus pass through the net, being dampened as it moved further from the source (Refs. 11.14, 11.15, and 11.16).

At present it is hard to know whether specificity for antigen or idiotype is the norm among suppressor T cells. Most of the evidence for anti-idiotype specificity comes from situations where antibody, i.e., a B cell product, does the suppressing, and we are more interested in knowing whether T cells can have such suppressor effects. There is a recent example in which administration of guinea pig anti-idiotype antibody to mice stimulated the appearance of suppressor T cells with the same anti-idiotype specificity; therefore, it seems that T cells can have this kind of activity. The interpretation of cases where suppressor T cells appear to be reacting against antigen are also complex (see below).

This brings us to a consideration of the mode and target of action of suppressor cells. It is impossible as yet to give a unifying account of suppressor mechanisms, or of helper effects, for that matter. There is an enormous body of recent research in the subject. One hopes that the mud will eventually settle to reveal a clear pool containing a few simple principles. It may be helpful to consider some possibilities, however. An apparently simple suppressor system is that illustrated in Table 11.2: suppressor cells against a protein will interfere with the cooperation between anti-protein helper T cells and anti-hapten B cells. Certain possible sites of action of a suppressor cell are shown in Fig. 11.3. The cellular interactions actually occurring *in vivo* must be much more complex than any such diagram can indicate. For example, R. K. Gershon (Ref. 11.13), a pioneer in the suppressor T cell field, has coined what he calls the second law of thymodynamics: "for every T cell-dependent augmentation there is an equal and opposite T cell suppression." This sort of generalization may prove to be a valuable way of summarizing the "logic" of suppression. It reflects his observation that, in many cases, a population of T cells activated to an antigen will suppress responses by other cells against the same antigen if these responses are already vigorous, but will augment them if they are weak. It seems probable that the cells being regulated provide some signals which affect the regulators, as well as the other way around.

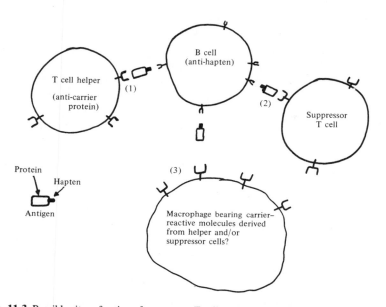

Fig. 11.3 Possible sites of action of suppressor T cells. (1) Against the idiotype of the helper cell receptors, (2) against the carrier determinants of the antigen, (3) competition with helper factors for space on the surface of a macrophage.

While the induction of either suppressor or helper T cells depends usually on contact with the specific antigen, it seems that many of the factors or signals which they produce are nonspecific, i.e., able to stimulate or depress other T and B cells of any specificity, provided these are nearby. The effect of linking two antigens, such as carrier protein and hapten, may be to "focus" these signals on to a second cell which is bound to another part of the same complex molecule. Experimental cases are, however, known where T cells responding to antigen X will enhance or suppress responses to an unlinked antigen Y. This suggests further levels of complexity of immune regulation. An important phenomenon which can probably be attributed to this kind of suppressor effect is *antigenic competition,* where the size of a response to antigen Y is decreased by prior or simultaneous injection of antigen X. The magnitude of such interference varies with different pairs of antigen, but it can make immunization with mixed vaccines undesirable.

We should note that "suppression" usually refers to the diminution of one particular class of specific immune response, e.g., IgG antibody formation; there may be no effect, or even an increase in other types of simultaneous activity, such as delayed-type hypersensitivity, against the same antigen. Very little is known about control of the class of immune reactions. Bretscher (Ref. 11.7) has recently introduced a scheme which explains many known facts, and is based on the idea that the level of available helper cells determines what class of response ensues: with few helpers, delayed hypersensitivity reactions occur, with progressively more, IgM and then IgG antibodies are made. There is evidence that suppression of antibody formation is sometimes accompanied by increased delayed hypersensitivity, a change which suppressor cells might bring about by regulating numbers of available helper cells. This question of class control is of great practical importance. For example, a delayed hypersensitivity reaction to a tumor may destroy it, while an IgG response may protect it (Section 14.3.4).

11.2.3 Self-Tolerance

A vitally important question for immunology is whether self-tolerance is maintained by active suppression, or by deletion of self-reactive cells. Obviously it is much more difficult to perform direct experiments on self-tolerance than on tolerance induced experimentally against a foreign antigen. For example, cell mixing experiments are only possible when one has a nontolerant population to mix with the tolerant one, and all lymphoid cell populations are normally self-tolerant.

Some logical arguments can, however, be adduced for suppressor self-tolerance:

1. Any new self-antigen which develops late (e.g., at puberty) should provoke an autoimmune reaction, since the immune repertoire should by this time include cells reactive against that antigen. Active suppression would be necessary to control such a reaction. Protagonists of deletion mechanisms in self-tolerance agree with this logical necessity, but argue that no entirely new self-antigens arise once the immune system is mature. The hormonal and other changes which occur in development may only involve increased production of antigens that were originally present in smaller amounts. It is hard to refute this. One instance of new self-antigens appearing late concerns the idiotypes of Ig, i.e., an immune response generates many new antibodies whose variable regions may appear to the animal producing them as novel antigens. This leads to the interesting "idiotype network" view of regulation as discussed above.

2. New immunocompetent cells are arising all the time, both from stem cells, and, some think, as variants within antigen-stimulated clones (Section 8.3.5). Many of these might be expected to react against self-antigens. While a majority could be deleted by a "one-hit" mechanism (Section 8.3.3), this seems a precarious mechanism on which to rely. Any local concentration of unexpurgated anti-self cells would start an autoimmune reaction, which, once started, would be impossible to stop except by suppressor means, since the self-antigens are obviously not removed.

3. The distinction between "self" and "not-self" antigens is not clear-cut.

There are thousands of self-antigens in a vertebrate, and many other antigens to which it can respond that must look very much like self. The suppressor view would be that an animal can make a response to something close to self only if this antigen appears at high concentration in lymphoid tissue. This response involves some transient autoimmune activity. Suppressor mechanisms control it, perhaps more rapidly and effectively if the antigen is similar to self.

In summary, arguments can be presented which predict that suppressor mechanisms will be found in self-tolerance. There is little direct evidence as yet: both deletion and suppression may well play a role. Reference 11.8 reviews the considerable evidence that anti-self-reactive cells do exist in normal animals, and describes an example of self-tolerance (to erythrocyte antigens) which seems to be maintained by active suppression.

11.2.4 Homogeneous Antibody

This chapter has stressed the degeneracy of the immune response, one manifestation of which is the variability between different individuals reacting against the same antigen. There are, however, certain antigens which provoke the synthesis of very restricted kinds of antibody that appear in all or most immunized animals. (Such cases figure prominently in the literature because they are often selected for study by immunochemists.) One good example is the small molecular weight compound phosphorylcholine. When this is coupled to any of a number of carriers and injected into, for example, a large group of outbred mice, most of the phosphorylcholine-specific antibody in each mouse will have the same idiotype; therefore, it probably has the same or closely similar primary structure in each case. Three explanations can be advanced for this:

1. The immune response is really a "determined" process after all; other cases where different animals make different antibodies reflect the fact that most antigens are heterogeneous and each animal is stimulated by, for example, hapten attached to slightly different molecular backgrounds. This is the extreme "chemical determinist" type of viewpoint.

2. There is a germline gene which codes for a V region with high affinity for phosphorycholine. Variants, therefore, have no selective advantage, and cells bearing the initial receptor predominate. This seems a possible explanation, but could become unlikely as examples of homogeneous antibody formation multiply, at least if one believes there are very few germline V genes.

3. For reasons of regulation, a particular idiotype has a selective advantage, e.g., this idiotype might be much more difficult to suppress than most others.

It is easy to see how one's general views on the immune system affect interpretation of phenomena like this. Several years ago point (3) would have seemed ridiculous. Now it seems a strong possibility.

11.3 GENETIC CONTROL OF IMMUNE RESPONSES

Any reaction as complex as the immune response must be affected by genetic factors. Some species are better than others at producing antibody against certain kinds of antigen, e.g., rabbits usually produce high-titer antibody to soluble proteins, while mice respond poorly to such antigens. Within species, strains which are systematically good or bad antibody producers have been developed by selective breeding. For example, Biozzi has produced two lines of mice which are "high" or "low" responders, respectively, to many antigens, and has estimated that at least ten genes play a role in such overall immune responsiveness.

In recent years, instances have been discovered where some genetic types in a species respond poorly or not at all to one particular antigen, while reacting normally against others. There seem to be two main types of specific immune response (Ir) genes responsible for these effects. First, there are genes in the Ig loci (Chapter 3) which control what particular antibody specificities or idiotypes animals make against certain antigens such as dextran or streptococcal polysaccharide (Ref. 3.8). While these cases are unusual in that they involve very homogeneous responses (and might therefore lead the sceptical to suspect some quirk of regulation), they are conventionally explained as reflecting the inheritance of particular immunoglobulin V genes. Second are a group of genes linked to the major histocompatibility complex (MHC); these form the subject of our subsequent discussion.

The first immune response gene of this latter kind was identified (by Benacerraf and colleagues) as determining the level of the antibody responses made by guinea pigs against a polypeptide containing only lysine residues. Subsequently, McDevitt, Benacerraf and others have found responses to at least forty different antigens which are influenced by Ir genes in mice. Similar genes occur in those other species so far examined, namely, guinea pigs, rats, monkeys, and probably in man. They are best demonstrated by immunizing under conditions which give a restricted response, that is, with low doses of antigens or with antigens which have a limited variety of different determinants, for example, a synthetic branched polypeptide polymer of tyrosine glutamic acid, alanine, and lysine, called (T,G)-A--L. It is said that large complex antigens induce antibodies of so many different specificities that genetic deficiencies in the response to any one determinant would be obscured.

11.3.1 The I Region of MHC

The property of non- (or low) responsiveness to various simple antigens has been shown to be genetically linked to the MHC. In most cases it appears, from back-cross experiments, that a single gene is involved, and in all instances, the gene is recessive, i.e., a cross between responder and nonresponder strains produces a heterozygote which is responsive. Only homozygous recessives are unresponsive. Without delving too deeply into the breeding experiments required (for which see Ref. 10.6), we can state that these Ir genes in mice are localized in one "I" region between K and SsSlp (Fig. 10.3). They are quite distinct from the histocompatibility K and D antigens discussed in Chapter 10. More recent mapping, following the segregation of several Ir genes among mice with recombinations within the MHC, has defined at least three subregions within I, namely, I-A, I-B, and I-C. (If individual mice are simultaneously nonresponders to more than one antigen, this implies that more than one gene is involved; the map has been built up from tests on several such strains.)

11.3.2 Functions of MHC-Linked Ir Genes

These Ir genes appear to affect cooperative interactions between cells. The genetic defects are expressed within the immunocompetent cells themselves: one can transfer responsiveness passively to irradiated nonresponder mice with responder cells. Several lines of evidence further suggest that the genes are expressed within T cells; while most studies on genetic unresponsiveness have measured antibody formation, cellular immunity to antigen, a characteristic T cell function, is also under Ir gene control; thymectomy abolishes antibody responses to antigens controlled by Ir genes; Ir genes are concerned with recognition and response to the carrier part of carrier–hapten conjugates, and, in fact, nonresponders to X may make anti-X antibody if stimulated with an XY conjugate, implying that only anti-X T cells, not B cells, were deficient; in agreement with this last observation, nonresponders have normal numbers of antigen binding B cells.

11.3.3 Ia Antigens

Having studied the function of Ir genes it was a natural next step to attempt to identify the gene products. The obvious procedure, for immunologists, was to immunize mice possessing one set of Ir genes with lymphocytes from mice with different Ir genes. Using many different strains of mice with known Ir phenotypes and known K and D alleles, it has been possible, by judicious cross-immunization and subsequent absorption of sera to produce specific anti-I region antisera. The antigens thus detected are called Ia antigens. Therefore, the I region of MHC contains Ir genes in several subregions whose presence influences the expression of Ia antigens. It is simplest to assume, although unproved, that the Ia antigens are actually coded for by the corresponding Ir genes.

These Ia antigens are glycoproteins which appear to exist on cells as complexes of two molecules of slightly different sizes, linked by disulfide bonds, and with a combined molecular weight of approximately 58,000. Like the K and D gene products, they are highly polymorphic; by late 1976, eighteen different antigenic specificities in the I-A subregion, and three in the I-C (although none in I-B) had been identified. Very recently, two further subregions, I-J and I-E, have been distinguished (Fig. 10.3). The Ia antigens are found on most B cells and on some T cells. They also occur on sperm, macrophages, and epithelial cells. Different immunocompetent cell types, it seems, may have I antigens from different subregions: thus B cells express I-A, I-E, and I-C antigens, and suppressor T cells I-J antigens (it is not yet known what subregion helper T cells display).

11.3.4 Factors Produced by T cells

T cells have been shown to produce a variety of factors which influence immune responses, factors which often contain Ia antigens. Many different experimental systems have been used in this work, often employing *in vitro* cultures of lymphocytes, and it would be fair to describe as unclear the relevance and interrelationships of these various T cell products to *in vivo* immune events. Some of the factors are specific, i.e., bind to a single antigen and influence responses to that antigen alone. Others are nonspecific. Some contain Ia antigens, while others do not, and some react with anti-Ig sera indicating that they have at least some part of an Ig molecule within their structure; others have no Ig component.

As concrete examples we can consider two of these factors. Taussig and Munro described an antigen-specific [anti-(T,G)-AL] helper factor, released by T cells, which was a glycoprotein of MW 50,000 and contained Ia antigens. The factor could be absorbed by B cells, and this absorption was prevented by pretreating the B cells with anti-Ia antisera, suggesting that two I region genes may be involved in T/B collaborative interactions: one for part of the T helper factor and another for some kind of acceptor molecule on B cells. A different, antigen-specific factor, also a 50,000 MW glycoprotein, was found by Tada in extracts from a population containing suppressor T cells. This carried antigen from the I-J subregion.

11.3.5 How Do the MHC-Linked Ir Genes Work?

If the Ia antigens are Ir gene products then it appears that Ir genes specify at least part of a molecule which is probably the T cell receptor. It was thought for a time that the Ir genes coded for the V region of such receptors, thus explaining the specificity of genetic unresponsiveness (absence of a gene). This seems less likely now if T cell receptors share idiotypes with B cell Ig (Section 9.2.1). It has also been suggested that the T cell receptor, which it sheds as a "factor," contains a V region from one of the Ig loci plus a C region which is Ia antigen; different Ia antigens might confer different properties on the specific molecule, e.g., helper or suppressor effects, much as the Fc piece of conventional Ig modulates the biological properties of the whole molecule. The difficulty with this idea, that Ir genes code for a ''constant'' region of T cell receptors, is that the specificity of Ir genes is left unexplained. A third possibility is that Ia antigens are not part of the T cell receptor, but in some way influence the repertoire of T cell specificities that develops during ontogeny. Two recent findings have made us aware that genetic control of immune responses is even more complex than it first appeared. There are at least two different I region genes involved in responses to some antigens and nonresponder animals in some cases do not lack immunocompetent cells but have specific suppressor cells.

11.3.6 Need for I Region Identity between Interacting Cells

T and B cells interact best if they both come from animals with the same I region genes. Similarly, there is a requirement for I region identity between macrophages and T cells in the generation of T helper cells. These phenomena are clearly analogous to the finding that cytotoxic T cells kill virus-infected target cells most efficiently if target and killer share K and D antigens (Section 9.4.5). A great deal of speculation has arisen out of these observations. For example, it has been argued that T cell receptors are genetically restricted to combining only with antigens coded for in the MHC regions or with closely related structures. As discussed in Section 9.4.5, this seems improbable: T cell receptors are likely to vary as widely and as randomly as B cell receptors. An apparently simple explanation for I region restriction is that helper cells become sensitized against a complex of exogenous antigen and adjacent Ia structures on a cell surface, and thereafter express a preference for cooperating with other cells of the same I region type which can reproduce the same complex on their surface. (Reference 9.5 develops this idea and refers to opposing points of view.)

11.3.7 Practical Importance of Ir Genes

Susceptibility to some diseases has been shown in both man and experimental animals to depend on genes of the MHC complex. For example, development of ragweed allergy in man (Section 12.2.3) depends on an HL-A-linked Ir gene that determines the production of IgE antibody against antigens of the plant. Certain HL-A types in man are associated with an increased incidence of a variety of diseases, and although possible reasons for this are complex (Ref. 11.18), linked Ir genes are probably involved in some cases. Increased knowledge of the function of the various genes in the MHC complex should have important repercussions in human and veterinary clinical medicine.

11.4 SUMMARY

A revolution appears to be underway in immunology. The old ideas of strictly determined, "all-or-none" responses are giving way to a view of the immune system as a complex network of interacting units. This chapter, while unavoidably vague in parts, has emphasized the current transitional nature of ideas in the subject.

It is first pointed out that immune responses are "degenerate," i.e., the same antigen provokes widely different responses in different animals. Reasons for this include the great complexity of immune induction, and the fact that any one antigen can stimulate quite a large proportion of the lymphocyte pool. This unpredictability of immune responses seems to demand that they be constantly regulated. Many cases of specific tolerance are now known to be maintained by active supression rather than by deletion of cells. The most important suppressor agents appear to be special kinds of T cell which may react specifically against either antigen or the idiotype of receptors on other cells responding to antigen. Some arguments for active suppression in self-tolerance are advanced.

The subsequent discussion of genetic control of immune responses centers around the immune response (Ir) genes present in the MHC complex of mice and other species. These genes affect responses to specific antigens by influencing cooperative cellular interactions. They seem to code for (Ia) antigens which are found on the surface of immunocompetent cells. T cells release a variety of factors which enhance or depress immune responses, and some of these factors are antigen specific and contain Ia antigens.

There are probably several "levels" of regulation of all immune responses. We have discussed two: the specific negative cellular influences which are common in tolerance and which may be generated during all immune responses and the genetically determined effect of certain MHC products on specific responses.

FURTHER READING

11.1   Allison, A. C., Denman, A. M., and Barnes, R. D. (1971). Cooperating and controlling functions of thymus-derived lymphocytes in relation to autoimmunity. *Lancet* **ii**, 135.

11.2   Asherson, G. L. and Zembala, M. (1975). Inhibitory T cells. *Curr. Topics Microbiol. Immunol.* **72**, 56.

11.3   Baker, P. J., Stashak, P. W., Amsbaugh, D. F., and Prescott, B. (1974). Regulation of the antibody response to type III pneumococcal polysaccharide. *J. Immunol.* **112**, 2020. An interesting and well-studied model system where tolerance is maintained by active suppression.

11.4   Basten, A., Miller, J. F. A. P., and Johnson, P. (1975). T cell-dependent suppression of an antihapten antibody response. *Transplant. Rev.* **26,** 130. (This volume of *Transplant. Rev.* contains several good articles about suppressor T lymphocytes.)

11.5   Benacerraf, B. (1974). Immune Response Genes. *Scand. J. Immunol.* **3,** 381. (A very clear, short review of this topic.)

11.6   Benacerraf, B. and Katz, D. H. (1975). The histocompatibility-linked immune response genes. *Adv. Cancer Res.* **21,** 121.

11.7   Bretscher, P. A. (1974). On the control between cell-mediated IgM and IgG immunity. *Cell. Immunol.* **13,** 171. A theory relating the class of immune response to the number of T helper cells available.

11.8   Cunningham, A. J. (1976). Self-tolerance maintained by active suppressor mechanisms. *Transplant. Rev.* **31,** 23.

11.9   Eardley, D. D., Staskawicz, M. O., and Gershon, R. K. (1976). Suppressor cells: dependence on assay conditions for functional activity. *J. Exp. Med.* **143,** 1211. Shows how the same population of activated T cells can have opposite effects on different populations of immunocompetent cells.

11.10   Eichmann, K. and Rajewsky, K. (1975). Induction of T and B cell immunity by anti-idiotype antibody. *Eur. J. Immunol.* **5,** 661. The use of anti-idiotype antibody to induce helper (or suppressor) T cells of the same specificity.

11.11   Feldmann, M. (1974). "Antigen specific T cell factors and their role in the regulation of T-B interaction. In "The Immune System; Genes, Receptors, Signals" (E. Sercarz, A. R. Williamson, and C. F. Fox, eds.), p. 497. Academic Press, New York. This volume also contains many other useful articles.

11.12   Fitch, F. W. (1975). Selective suppression of immune responses. *Progr. Allergy* **19,** 195. Mainly about anti-idiotype regulation.

11.13   Gershon, R. K. (1974). T cell control of antibody production. *Contemp. Top. Immunobiol.* **3,** 1.

11.14   Jerne, N. K. (1973). The immune system. *Sci. Am.* **229,** 52. An account written for the layman, and introducing the network idea.

11.15   Jerne, N. K. (1974). Towards a network theory of the immune system. *Ann. Immunol. (Paris)* **125C,** 373.

11.16   Lindenmann, J. (1973). "Speculation on idiotypes and homobodies." *Ann. Immunol. (Paris).* **124C,** 171. A very clear exposition of the idiotype network idea.

11.17   McCullagh, P. (1972). The abrogation of immunological tolerance by means of allogeneic confrontation. *Transplant. Rev.* **12,** 180. A review by a pioneer of the concept that tolerance may be maintained by suppression rather than deletion.

11.18   Munro, A. and Bright, S. (1976). Products of the major histocompatibility complex and their relationship to the immune response. *Nature (London)* **264,** 145. A very clear review.

11.19   Scibienski, R. J., Harris, L. M., Fong, S., and Benjamini, E. (1974). Active and inactive states of immunologic unresponsiveness. *J. Immunol.* **113,** 45.

11.20   Strayer, D. S., Lee, W. M. F., Rowley, D. A., and Kohler, H. (1975). Anti-receptor antibody. II. Induction of long-term unresponsiveness in neonatal mice. *J. Immunol.* **114,** 728. An example of a relatively homogeneous response (to phosphorylcholine), inhibited by anti-idiotype antisera.

11.21   Voisin, G. A. (1971). Immunity and tolerance: a unified concept. *Cell. Immunol.* **2,** 670. A review by one of the first workers to realize that immunity and tolerance may both be disturbances of regulation.

11.22   Waksman, B. H. and Namba, Y. (1976). On soluble mediators of immunologic regulation. *Cell. Immunol.* **21,** 161.

QUESTIONS

11.1 A biochemist friend of yours has three different proteins, A, B, and C. He prepares antisera against A by injecting it into four rabbits, then tests the sera, with an antigen binding assay, against each of the three proteins. He obtains the following results:

Antiserum from rabbit	Serum titers against protein.		
	A	B	C
1	1/16,000	1/4,000	1/250
2	1/32,000	1/2,000	1/500
3	1/16,000	1/16,000	1/500
4	1/4,000	1/8,000	1/100

Your friend, whose ideas on immunology are essentially those current at the time of Landsteiner, is alarmed by the fact that the different individual rabbits do not "see" the same relationship between the three proteins.* In particular he is worried about rabbit 4, because this one produced a higher titer against a protein other than the immunizing antigen. How would you reassure your friend, and what conclusions about A, B, and C would you draw from the experiment?

11.2 According to conventional views, immune responses are specific because the antigen *selects*, from a diverse preexisting array of immunocompetent cells, only a tiny proportion whose receptors have relatively high affinity for that antigen. Certain recent evidence suggests, however, that a single antigen may stimulate a large proportion of lymphocytes (Section 11.1). If this were true, what questions would it raise about the specificity of immune reactions? (This problem is difficult, controversial, and lies at the "growing edge" of immunology. It may help to think back to Chapter 1.)

*No reference to any particular biochemist, either living or dead, is intended here!

Aberrations of the Immune System: Immune Deficiency, Allergy, and Autoimmune Disease

Many of the functions of the immune system can be harmful. For example, a severe delayed hypersensitivity reaction may cause local tissue damage. Rejection of a kidney allograft may cost the life of a patient. Yet one would not want to class these immune activities as aberrant. Delayed hypersensitivity reactions are valuable in preventing the spread of infectious organisms (Section 9.4.3). Grafts are rejected because it is the normal function of the immune system to react against foreign material. It is the situation which is artificial. These kinds of activity may also be important in the destruction of tumors (Chapter 14).

There are, however, three kinds of clinical conditions which it seems fair to classify as aberrations of immune function. The first is the diverse group of immune deficiency diseases where lymphocytes or immunoglobulins are deficient or absent. The second are the allergic conditions mediated by antibody. These may have some protective effects (see below) but at present they appear to do more harm than good. Finally, there are a variety of autoimmune diseases, caused by breakdown of self-tolerance.

12.1 IMMUNOLOGICAL DEFICIENCY DISEASES

One of the practical benefits of the dissection of the immune system into its components by modern immunological research has been a greatly improved understanding of human immune deficiency states. These include an array of disorders which may lie in the stem cells themselves, or in the inductive micro-environments which allow differentiation of more mature lymphocytes, or in the final balance of cell populations needed for regulation of effector cells. Apart from some rare abnormalities of phagocytes, they may be classified into two groups, representing failure of T or B systems, respectively.

The first immune deficiency state identified (in 1952) was Bruton's disease: infantile, X-linked *hypogammaglobulinemia*. Serum IgG levels are low in this condition (about 1 mg/ml), while IgA and IgM are virtually absent. B lymphocytes are missing from blood and secondary lymphoid tissue, and antibody responses are, not surprisingly, very poor. Cell-mediated immune functions are, however, normal. More common than Bruton's disease are a variety of B lymphocyte maturation defects, in which surface Ig-bearing lymphocytes themselves may exist although serum Ig levels and antibody responses are very low. Possible causes of such syndromes include intrinsic defects of the B lymphocytes or failures of cooperation between T and B cells. There have been intriguing recent reports that certain hypogammaglobulinemias may be caused by abnormalities of suppressor T cells; the synthesis of Ig by normal peripheral blood lymphocytes cultured *in vitro* with a mitogen (Section 9.1.3) was suppressed when lymphocytes from hypogammaglobulinemic patients were added to the cultures.

The most extreme T cell defect known in man is DiGeorge's syndrome, caused by a developmental failure of the thymus (and parathyroid glands). There are few or no T cells, and cell-mediated immunity is defective. However, while the anatomical defect in these patients is comparable to that in nude or neonatally thymectomized mice, their ability to make antibody is only marginally affected. This may indicate that some T cell function can develop during fetal life under the influence of thymic hormone from the mother, an idea which is supported by the recent experimental observation that nude mouse offspring of normal mothers make much better antibody responses than nude mice born to mothers who were themselves without a thymus.

Combined T and B cell deficiencies are also known in humans, where they are an important cause of death in the early postnatal years. In severe cases, there are few lymphocytes of either kind in blood or lymphoid tissue. A classification of human immune deficiency states may be found in Ref. 12.4. The impact of such deficiencies on resistance to infectious disease is further discussed in Chapter 13.

12.2 ALLERGIC OR HYPERSENSITIVITY REACTIONS

12.2.1 Terminology

Both terminology and phenomena in this area are rather confusing. "Allergy" was originally coined to describe any state of altered responsiveness induced by prior exposure to antigen, i.e., immunological memory. Increased resistance was called "immunity" and increased susceptibility to antigenic challenge (e.g.,

TABLE 12.1
Classification of Principal Hypersensitivity States

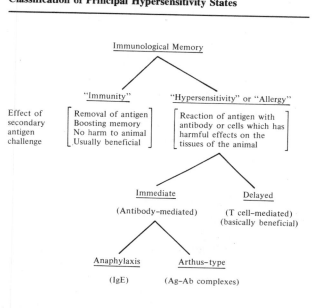

with a toxin) was termed "hypersensitivity." Current usage is summarized in Table 12.1. We can consider "hypersensitivity" or "allergy" as synonymous terms for a particular class of memory states in which antigen challenge causes damage to the host. These hypersensitivity states fall into two distinct categories: those mediated by T cells which, as we have seen (Section 9.4.1), are characterized by *delayed* reactions to injection of antigen into the skin (24 hours or more); and those mediated by free antibody, which are called *"immediate"* because skin challenge gives much more rapid local reactions (within a period ranging from a few minutes to about 8 hours). The term "allergy" is now usually applied to potentially harmful states of antibody mediated immediate hypersensitivity, although there have been attempts by some to revive its older meaning as describing any immune memory state.

12.2.2 Immediate Hypersensitivity

Antibodies produced in response to prior contact with an antigen can, on subsequent challenge with the antigen, prove harmful rather than beneficial under two main sets of circumstances: (1) when a particular type of antibody, IgE, predominates causing "anaphylactic" sensitivity (Fig. 12.1); and (2) when antibody and antigen are present in such large amounts in the blood that complexes form in the tissues and provoke local inflammation.

12.2.3 Anaphylactic Sensitivity

Portier and Richet, in 1902, immunized a dog against the poison of a sea anemone; when reinjected some weeks later with the same antigen, the dog died suddenly with symptoms of shock. "Anaphylaxis" is the term coined by these workers (from the Greek "ana," against, and "phylaxis," protection), to mean the opposite of "prophylaxis," and to dramatize the fact that the consequences of immune reactions could be harmful. It was later shown, by Prausnitz and Kustner, in 1921, that a state of anaphylactic sensitivity could be passively transferred with serum. The serum substance responsible was called "reagin."

Because it is present in such small amounts in human serum (average concentration about 100 ng/ml), the identification of reagin as a new class of immunoglobulin, IgE, has been achieved only recently. The structure of the ϵ chain (Section 3.2) has now been worked out from myeloma proteins of this class. The Fc portion of the ϵ chain binds to specific receptor sites, many thousands of which occur on the plasma membranes of mast cells and basophil polymorphonuclear leukocytes. These cells have large cytoplasmic granules; when antigen binds to, and cross-links, cytophilic IgE molecles on the surface of a mast cell (Fig. 12.1), a conformational change occurs in the membrane, which in turn leads to release of histamine and other vasoactive amines (serotonin, kinins, "slow-reactive substance"), from the cytoplasmic granules. These substances cause contraction of smooth muscle, and dilation and increased permeability of small blood vessels, effects which give rise to the symptoms of anaphylactic shock. If an individual has specific IgE antibody attached to mast cells in the respiratory tract, the symptoms after inhaling the antigen will be sneezing, and wheezing, with respiratory failure in severe cases. If the antigen is injected into the skin and encounters antibody attached to mast cells there, cutaneous anaphylaxis results, a rapid local reddening and swelling which reaches peak intensity in about 30 minutes. Thus cutaneous reaction is used to diagnose the hypersensitive state, by rubbing, into a scratch on a patient's skin, a little of the antigen to which it is suspected that he is sensitive.

Just what conditions favor the production of IgE over other Ig classes is unclear. Experimental animals (and humans) can become "sensitized" by a single initial injection of soluble protein antigens intravenously, intraperitoneally, or intradermally. It seems probable that prolonged contact with certain antigens at mucous surfaces or on the skin may lead to sensitization, e.g., grass pollen in the respiratory tract, some species of helminths in the gut. Note that a state of "sensitivity" in this context denotes the presence of circulating and mast cell-attached IgE with specificity for a particular antigen: on challenge with that

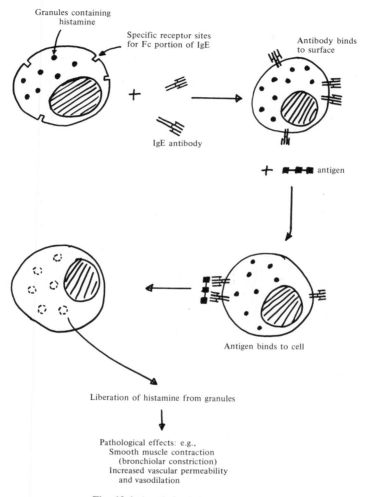

Fig. 12.1 Anaphylactic hypersensitivity.

antigen, an immediate reaction occurs. This is a memory state in the broad sense, but is different in principle from the memory carried by increased numbers of specific lymphocytes able to react with antigen and make more Ig over a period of days.

Among humans, some ("atopic") individuals have a propensity toward developing relatively high levels of IgE and hence anaphylactic sensitivities against extrinsic "allergens" such as grass pollen, mites in house dust, animal dandruff, some foods (e.g., strawberries, shellfish), insect bites, and some drugs (e.g., penicillin). Such atopic tendencies are strongly inherited. Other species make IgE-like molecules, and some, like the mouse and the guinea pig, also have IgG_1 molecules with *homocytotropic* (cell-sticking) properties which can contribute to anaphylactic reactions.

The determined reader who, undismayed by terms like "reagin," "homocytotropic," and "atopy," advances further into the relevant literature, will soon encounter some cumbersome new expressions, two of which deserve mention here. "Passive cutaneous anaphylaxis" is a test for serum IgE: suspect serum is injected intradermally into a normal animal of the same species, where IgE fixes to skin mast cells; several hours later a challenge dose of antigen is given intravenously, together with Evans blue dye; local skin reactions cause increased capillary permeability with uptake of dye as a visible patch. The "Prausnitz–Kustner" reaction is similar, except that the antigen is not injected intravenously, but into the same area as the IgE-containing serum, where it causes local reaction.

Treatment of these allergies is usually symptomatic, e.g., with antihistamines. A specific immunological treatment is sometimes attempted: repeated and gradually increasing doses of the allergen may "desensitize," perhaps by causing helper T cells to become tolerant, or by diverting the immune response into production of an alternative class of immunoglobulin, such as IgG, which does not bind to mast cells. Recently, there has been an exciting new finding: the synthetic pentapeptide, Asp-Ser-Asp-Pro-Arg, which resembles a region characteristic of the ϵ chain Fc region, has been shown to block Fc binding sites on mast cells, partially inhibiting subsequent specific anaphylactic reactions. Clearly, such blocking agents could potentially prevent the development of anaphylactic sensitivity.

Anaphylactic reactions have historically been regarded as a serious nuisance, hence their inclusion in this chapter. However, it is increasingly thought that they may have useful functions as well. For example, some gut worms may induce a local proliferation of mast cells which become sensitized with specific IgE and, after binding to antigens of the parasites, release substances contributing to its expulsion. The fact that IgE has been retained by evolution, and the abundance of mast cells in mucosal areas, suggest an important physiological role for IgE, perhaps in preventing infections at such surfaces. Anaphylaxis may prove to be simply an undesirable side effect of a basically protective process.

12.2.4 Arthus-Type Sensitivity

This is also an antibody dependent allergic state, but of quite a different type from anaphylactic hypersensitivity. When very high levels of precipitating antibody of any class exist in the circulation, then a localized injection of the specific antigen can cause formation of antigen–antibody precipitates which are deposited in blood vessel walls. A variety of secondary effects may follow. There is an acute inflammatory reaction, with infiltration of polymorphonuclear leukocytes. Complement may be fixed and/or platelets aggregated with subsequent release of vasoactive substances. The reaction differs from anaphylaxis and from delayed hypersensitivity responses in several ways: IgE is not required; a cutaneous reaction is much slower (peaking at 4–8 hours) than cutaneous anaphylaxis, although still considerably faster than a delayed hypersensitivity reaction; and a polymorph infiltration is characteristic, in contrast to the mononuclear infiltrates of delayed (T cell) reactions and to the relative lack of cellular infiltration in anaphylaxis.

The clinical picture is said to depend on the *relative* amounts of antigen and antibody involved. If antibody predominates, antigen is precipitated at the site of injection. In antigen excess, smaller soluble complexes may be disseminated around the body causing lesions in joints, skin, kidneys, and lymphatic tissue. This latter kind of syndrome is seen in *serum sickness,* brought about by therapeutic injections of, for example, very large amounts of horse anti-tetanus immunoglobulin. This foreign protein can persist in the circulation until anti-horse Ig antibody appears 1–2 weeks later, when precipitates may form with the horse Ig.

Arthus reactions can be regarded as an exaggerated form of the normal clearance of antigen by circulating antibody. They probably have no beneficial effects. Other kinds of hypersensitivity state are distinguished by some authors. There is a more detailed account in Roitt's textbook, for example (Ref. 1.5).

12.3 AUTOIMMUNE DISEASE

There are a great variety of pathological conditions caused by immune reactions against self-components. In some of these, only a single organ is affected: Hashimoto's disease involves mononuclear cell infiltration of the thyroid gland and autoantibody production against certain of its constituents; in pernicious anemia the target is "instrinsic factor" which normally mediates vitamin B_{12} absorption, but may be prevented from doing so by autoantibody; certain hemolytic anaemias can be caused by autoantibody which destroys erythrocytes. At the other end of the scale are diseases in which the damage is diffused through many tissues. The paradigm is *systemic lupus erythematosus* (SLE) in which antibodies are made to DNA and other constituents of cell nuclei. Antigen–antibody complexes form which localize in many tissues, skin, joints, lymph nodes, spleen, liver, lung, gastrointestinal tract, and particularly in the kidneys. The disease has features in common with serum sickness (Section 12.2.4), presumably because in both cases it is the abnormal accumulation of complexes which is damaging; but whereas serum sickness quickly resolves itself, as the antigen disappears, SLE persists usually for the lifetime of the patient (years) since the responsible self-antigens are indispensable. Other examples of human disease with autoimmune etiology are: Addison's disease, rheumatoid arthritis, some infertilities, myasthenia gravis (recently attributed to autoantibody formation against the acetylcholine receptor at neuromuscular junctions), and some types of diabetes. New candidates come under suspicion from time to time, e.g., schizophrenia. A more complete list is given by Rose in Ref. 1.6.

Other important facts about autoimmunity are the following:

1. Many clinically normal individuals have low titers of antibody against some of their own tissues, e.g., against erythrocytes. Thus, autoimmune activity is not in itself abnormal. It is dangerous only if too vigorous.

2. A related point is that autoantibodies are more common in older people than in young.

3. Women are more prone to autoimmune disease than men.

4. Genetic factors are clearly involved in autoimmune disease: there is strong tendency for it to run in families (this is also true of allergies). Breeding studies with autoimmune experimental animals (NZB mice, below) have shown that several different genes are important.

5. Affected individuals often have more than one autoimmune disorder, suggesting that the basic lesion may be an increased tendency to react against any self-antigen.

6. Antibodies are causative agents in may of these diseases. The role of cell-mediated autoimmunity is less clear, but the mononuclear cell infiltrates seen in organ-specific autoimmune disease suggests that T cells may also be reacting against self.

12.3.1 Experimental Models

Injection of isologous organ extracts in complete Freund's adjuvant will often provoke autoimmune activity against the corresponding organ. Thus rabbit thyroglobulin can induce thyroiditis in rabbits; injections of emulsified brain can induce encephalitis in monkeys and guinea pigs.

Some strains of experimental animals have been produced in which autoimmune disease appears regularly and spontaneously. The best known is the NZB (New Zealand Black) mouse. These animals consistently develop, at several months of age, an autoimmune hemolytic anemia. They have a positive Coombs' test, that is, their erythrocytes become coated with antibody which does not in itself agglutinate them, but these erythrocytes can be agglutinated *in vitro* by adding antibody to mouse globulin (Section 2.2.5).

12.3.2 Causes of Autoimmune Disease

As one might expect, there is a stimulating amount of disagreement about the causes of autoimmune disease. Ideas fall into two main groups (Table 12.2). The first approach is to blame everything on the environment: extrinsic agents such as mechanical damage or infectious organisms alter the availability or presentation of self-antigens which then become immunogenic. The oldest notion was that autoimmune reactions are only directed against normally hidden or "sequestered" self-components, that is, tissues like brain, lens, and testis which lie outside the lymphocyte recirculation pathway, or against normally hidden components of other organs released by damage. This idea is no longer tenable. For example, red cells surface antigens are available to the developing immune system, and small amounts of thyroglobulin circulate in serum, yet autoantibodies can be made against both of these self-antigens. However, the newer idea that "altered presentation" of antigens is responsible for breakdown of self-tolerance has quite wide support (Fig. 12.2). One could imagine that all T cells with self-reactivity were deleted (this has not been proved), while anti-self B cells were retained, but could not be stimulated for lack of T help. Coupling a self-antigen to a new carrier might enable a bypass of this tolerance by employing T cells reactive to foreign antigens (Fig. 12.2). This could occur with virus-infected cells, for example, with the virus serving as a carrier. As a concrete example, autoimmunity to heart muscle in rheumatic fever is believed to be induced in response to a constituent of group A streptococci that cross-reacts with heart antigen. Emulsification of self-components in Freund's adjuvant may also produce such hybrid self-foreign complexes. Alternatively, a foreign antigen may possess both foreign determinants and others which resemble self-antigens of the animal to which it gains access.

The second group of ideas on autoimmunity (not necessarily exclusive of the first) is that some failure of the lymphoid system is the precipitating cause. This

TABLE 12.2
Possible Causes of Autoimmune Disease

Cause	Mechanism	Type of tolerance implied
1. Extrinsic agents	Damage to organ, release of sequestered antigens	No tolerance against normally sequestered antigens
	Cross-reacting environmental agents (T tolerance circumvented)	Deletion of cells reactive to self-components
2. Abnormality of Immune function	Forbidden clone (mutant)	Deletion
	Failure of suppression	Suppressor tolerance

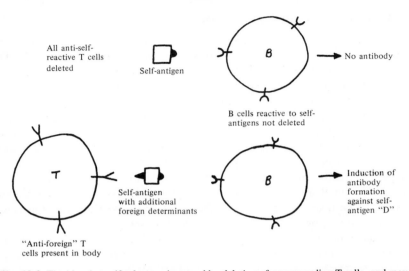

Fig. 12.2 The idea that self-tolerance is caused by deletion of corresponding T cells, and may be broken by immunizing with an antigen which has foreign antigenic determinants coupled to self-components.

theory divides again into two very different subgroups (Table 12.2). The older Burnetian view was, as we saw in Section 8.3.1, that self-tolerance is established early in life, but that mutant ''forbidden'' clones may arise later and cause damage. The more recent view of some immunologists would be that self-tolerance is a failure of suppression, a failure adequately to control autoimmune reactions which are perhaps always proceeding at a low level in normal individuals.

As Table 12.2 shows, we can also classify the possible causes of autoimmunity according to whether we believe that self-tolerance is normally maintained by deletion or suppression. A failure of deletion tolerance as the cause of autoimmune disease is invoked both by the ''forbidden clone'' concept and by the idea that extrinsic agents bypass an absolute self-tolerance in T cells. For suppressor self-tolerance there is little direct experimental support as yet, although there are some intriguing indications: lymphatic leukemia is often associated with autoimmune disease, suggesting that an immune control mechanism has been impaired by the lymphocyte disorder; autoimmune diseases occur in groups in single individuals also suggesting a control lesion; recent experiments have shown that thymus cells (suppressors?) from young NZB mice may diminish the hemolytic disease when injected into older NZB mice. A reasonably conservative view at the moment would be that there may be deletion of most immunocompetent cells reactive against those self-components which are present in large amounts. Extrinsic agents like cross-reacting antigens no doubt stimulate bursts of autoimmunity, but it seems likely that in normal individuals, these episodes are prevented from escalating by suppressor control mechanisms. A more radical view would be that self-tolerance is a balance between cells which can react against self-antigen and an equally powerful cohort of suppressor cells, which prevent them from doing so.

12.4 SUMMARY

This chapter briefly describes three groups of conditions in which immune functions are lacking or mainly harmful in their consequences for the host.

1. Immune deficiency diseases fall into two principal groups, reflecting impaired activity of T or B cell lines.

2. Immediate hypersensitivity reactions are caused by antibody, in previously sensitized animals, which reacts immediately and in a damaging way with specific challenge antigen. The two most important examples are: first, anaphylactic sensitivity, where IgE is cytophilically bound to mast cells in various tissues and subsequently combines with antigen releasing vasoactive amines from the mast cell cytoplasmic granules; and second, Arthus sensitivity, in which high circulating concentrations of precipitating antibody form, with challenge antigen, complexes which are deposited in blood vessel walls initiating acute local inflammatory reactions.

3. Autoimmune diseases involve reactions against self-antigens. Current ideas about causes fall into two main groups: (a) that self-reactive (T) cells are deleted, but autoimmunity can be induced by altering self-antigens in such a way that existing T cells of other specificities can recognize them and stimulate a response; (b) that autoimmune reactions are a result of the failure of normal suppressor self-tolerance mechanisms.

FURTHER READING

12.1   Allison, A. C. (1974). The roles of T and B lymphocytes in self-tolerance and autoimmunity. *Contemp. Top. Immunobiol.* **3,** 227.

12.2   Bretscher, P. A. (1973). A model for generalized autoimmunity. *Cell. Immunol.* **6,** 1. An explanation for autoimmune disease based on the Bretscher/Cohn theory of self-tolerance.

12.3   Burnet, F. M. (1972). "Autoimmunity and Autoimmune Disease." F. A. Davis Co., Philadelphia, Pennsylvania.

12.4   Cooper, M. D., Faulk, W. P., Fudenberg, H. H., Good, R. A., Hitzig, W., Kunkel, H. G., Roitt, I. M., Rosen, F. S., Seligmann, M., Soothill, J. F., and Wedgewood, R. J. (1974). Primary immunodeficiencies. Meeting Report of the 2nd International Workshop on Primary Immunodeficiency Diseases in May. *Clin. Immunol. Immunopathol.* **2,** 416.

12.5   Fudenberg, H. *et al.* (1971). Primary immunodeficiencies. *Pediatrics* **47**, 927.

12.6   Hamburger, R. N. (1976). Allergy and the immune system. *Am. Sci.* **64**, 157. A simple account of IgE and its effects.

12.7   Ishizaka, T. and Ishizaka, K. (1975). Regulation of reaginic antibody formation in animals. *Prog. Allergy* **19**, 122.

12.8   Moller, G. (ed.). (1976). Autoimmunity and self-nonself discrimination. *Transplant. Rev.* **31**. A collection of papers on this topic.

12.9   Turk, J. L. (1973). "Immunology in Clinical Medicine." Heinmann, London. Mostly about the harmful effects of immune reactions.

QUESTIONS

12.1   The author, who has been experimenting with mice for some years, now gets various disagreeable symptoms if he enters a room where mice are caged. Among these symptoms are a certain wheezing and difficulty in breathing which appears after about 20 minutes. What causes this? What would happen if a mouse bit the author, or rubbed itself against a scratch on his hand?

12.2   Virus infection of cells can lead to the appearance of new (virus-specified) antigens on the surface of these cells. Explain how a virus infection of, say, muscle cells might provoke production of autoantibodies against normal muscle constituents (see Fig. 12.2 if necessary).

Immunity to Infectious Disease

Many organisms live on or inside the bodies of others. This association is by no means always harmful to the host: for example, bacteria in the gut of ruminants digest cellulose into sugars which the mammal can then metabolize; the skin and mucous membranes of vertebrates support many normally harmless species of bacteria and fungi. Such organisms which do little or no damage to their hosts are, in an ecological sense, the most successful of parasites since they do not endanger the supply of their preferred "habitat." Many other parasites, by contrast, cause a variety of disease states, ranging from the chronic debilitation induced by blood-sucking helminths, which may remain in one host for years, to the rapidly developing infections brought about by some viruses and bacteria which may sweep through a susceptible species in weeks.

In evolutionary terms, both hosts and parasites seek to survive and propagate their kind. Vertebrates will slowly evolve, over many generations, to acquire "natural" resistance against pathogenic invaders. However, the enormous numbers and rapid generation times of most parasites, particularly microorganisms, allow them to produce new and virulent genetic variants much faster than their vertebrate hosts can change to resist them. It was probably to counter the constant threat of such "unexpected" (Chapter 1) infectious organisms that vertebrates developed an immune system, and the science of immunology has grown out of a practical desire to understand and exploit immune defense mechanisms. Evolutionary aspects of immunity are further discussed in Chapter 15; in this section we will examine what is known about immunity against infection.

13.1 IMMUNE MECHANISMS

The importance of immune mechanisms to infectious disease is demonstrated by two kinds of observations: first, that individuals who have recovered from a disease are usually immune to reinfection, and second, that people lacking some part of their immune system are often disastrously prone to infections. The first observation has been a part of human scientific knowledge for thousands of years, while the second comes from the application of immunological ideas to modern medicine. Thus, people with hypogammaglobulinemia, abnormally low levels of gamma-globulin in their serum (Section 12.1), have very low resistance to bacterial infections although their immunity to most viruses develops normally. Patients with leukopenia (low numbers of circulating leukocytes), but with normal levels of antibody, are likewise liable to severe bacterial infections. Children lacking a thymus can cope with common bacterial infections but have deficient cell-mediated immunity (see below) and may be killed by such viruses as vaccinia and measles, or by BCG (Chapter 9) tuberculosis vaccine.

It is usual to divide immune resistance to disease into "innate" and "acquired" mechanisms (Table 13.1). Acquired immunity embraces all of the processes discussed in the rest of this book. Under "innate" resistance may be grouped a variety of usually nonspecific factors and features of the general physiology of animals which do not depend on specific immunization, but which contribute to their resistance to infectious disease. While innate immunity is perhaps not strictly part of immunology it deserves some discussion, since the mechanisms are clinically very important. Many of them act in concert with

TABLE 13.1
Principal Innate and Acquired Immune Resistance Mechanisms

Resistance mechanism	Agent
Innate	Genetic and physiological factors
	Humoral agents
	Secretions on skin and mucous membranes
	Interferon
	Natural antibody (acquired?)
	Complement
	Phagocytic cells
	Polymorphonuclear leukocytes
	Macrophages
Acquired	Antibody
	Neutralization of toxins or infective agents
	Lysis of bacteria and infected cells
	Recruitment (+antigen) of phagocytic cells
	Sensitization for opsonization
	Sensitization for K cell killing
	Cell-mediated immunity
	T cells
	Cytotoxic
	Lymphokine producing
	Activated macrophages

specific, adaptive immune processes, and in fact resistance to most diseases depends on the complex interplay of many mechanisms, both innate and acquired.

13.1.1 Innate Resistance

13.1.1.1 *"Genetic" and physiological factors*

Different species vary in their susceptibility to different parasites, for reasons which are usually unknown. Men and guinea pigs contract diphtheria, while rats are resistant. Within species there are often marked strain differences, e.g., American Indians and Negroes are much more susceptible to tuberculosis than are Caucasians. In experimental animals some genetic differences in resistance are known to be caused by differences in Ir gene inheritance (Section 11.3.7). Diet can affect resistance; starvation increases susceptibility to bacterial infections. The influence of hormones on disease resistance and immune responses has been surprisingly little studied, but must be significant, e.g., cortisone decreases phagocytosis and antibody formation.

13.1.1.2 *Humoral agents*

A variety of nonspecific agents seem to have been evolved for the specialized function of resisting potentially invasive organisms. On the skin, lactic acid in sweat and fatty acids in sebaceous secretions kill many bacteria and fungi. The mucus of respiratory and genital tracts is bacteriocidal and virucidal. An important defense mechanism against viruses is the release, within hours, of *interferon* by infected cells. This is a protein which prevents intracellular replication of the invading virus or of different viruses. The so-called "natural antibodies" are important in defense against some bacteria or viruses; by contrast with the above agents, these are *specific* immunoglobulins, usually IgM, which exist in small amounts in animals not known to have had contact with the particular pathogen studied. It is likely that they are provoked by cross-reacting antigens or by mitogens from the environment (e.g., in food, dust, or gut flora), in which case they should perhaps be classified as an acquired rather than innate resistance mechanism. Antibodies in newborn animals derived from the mother across the placenta or through the milk present a similar difficulty of classification but are often very important in conferring (passive) resistance on the young (Section 2.4).

13.1.1.3 *Phagocytic cells*

Both mononuclear and polymorphonuclear phagocytes (Section 4.2.4) are induced to congregate in inflamed sites by substances released by invading bacteria or by damaged cells. Particles that become attached to the plasma

membranes of phagocytes are engulfed and often destroyed as cytoplasmic lyso-
somes fuse with and discharge their hydrolytic enzymes into the phagocytic
vacuoles. This kind of protection is not infallible, however, since some viruses,
rickettsia, protozoa, and exceptionally hardy bacteria such as *Brucella* and
Mycobacterium tuberculosis can survive or multiply inside phagocytic cells.

   How do phagocytes discriminate between foreign particles, which they ingest,
and self-components, which they normally leave alone? In the case of vertebrate
phagocytes this recognition problem is often solved by allowing specific antibody to do the discriminating. Phagocytosis is greatly assisted by a group of
serum substances collectively called "opsonins" (after the Greek "opsono": I
prepare food for), which include some antibodies and complement (Fig. 13.1).
Antibodies are often available against foreign but not self-antigens. Anything to
which antibody combines will be readily phagocytized. Thus foreign material is
ingested, while normal self-components are not. (It is interesting to note that
degenerating self-components, such as old red cells, *are* often phagocytized,
after first becoming coated with antibody against new antigenic determinants
revealed during the degeneration process.) This relegation of self/not self deci-
sions to antibody is conceptually satisfying, but unfortunately cannot fully explain the behavior of phagocytes, since invertebrates which have no antibody
also contain phagocytic cells that do not attack their "hosts." Some other more

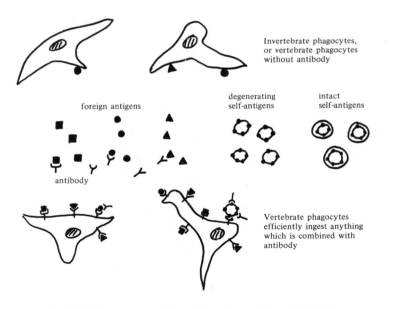

Fig. 13.1 Phagocytosis, with or without the assistance of antibody.

primitive way of distinguishing foreign objects must exist, although one would not expect this to have the same power as the vertebrate immune system to detect fine differences in chemical composition. It is likely that vertebrate phagocytes also retain some ability to ingest particles in the absence of antibody, albeit much less efficiently, although there is disagreement about this: it is difficult to prove that there is absolutely no specific antibody attached initially either to the antigen or to the surface of the phagocyte ("cytophilic" antibody, see below).

The role of phagocytic cells in immunity was the subject of violent controversy for many years. Eli Metchnikoff, a Russian biologist who in 1882 observed phagocytosis of foreign particles by scavenger cells in starfish, championed the view that this kind of mechanism alone could explain resistance to invasion by microorganisms. This was hotly contested by German workers at the Pasteur Institute in Paris, who felt that humoral factors were all important. As often happens in scientific disputes, it now seems that the truth lies between these extremes: both phagocytes and antibody are vital, and they may function cooperatively.

13.1.1.4 Complement, and other auxilliary substances

Complement (abbreviated C') is a series of eleven protein components in normal serum which are involved in such defense mechanisms as opsonization, local inflammation, and lysing bacteria and cells. These proteins are normally inert, but can be activated in a complex sequential reaction analogous to the blood clotting mechanism. In (simplified) outline, the process is as follows. The first stage of activation is provoked by combination of antigen with IgM or IgG antibody, which causes a conformational change in the normal Fc structure of the immunoglobulin leading to binding of the first component of complement, C1. This bound C1 now acquires the ability to activate several molecules of the next component in the chain, which, in turn, act on the next in enzymatic fashion, one molecule triggering many in a self-amplifying cascade. The process is controlled by a series of inhibitors. At certain stages, fragments with pharmacological activities are split off the complement molecules, for example, "anaphylatoxins" which promote histamine release, and other fragments which are chemotactic for granulocytes (i.e., encourage their local accumulation). The end result of the complement cascade initiated by antibody attached to antigen on a cell surface is the activation of terminal components which can punch a microscopically visible hole in the membrane causing lysis of the cell or bacterium. In Chapters 2 and 4 we discussed how this property of complement is used in serum and plaque forming cell tests for hemolytic antibody.

Active intermediates of the complement sequence can be induced, not only by antigen–antibody complexes as in the "classical pathway" outlined above, but also by an "alternate pathway," stimulated by certain bacterial cell wall polysaccharides, such as endotoxin. *Properdin* is a 230,000 molecular weight protein in normal serum which is involved in this alternate pathway of complement activation. *Immunoconglutinin* is an autoantibody against new antigenic determinants which are revealed when complement binds to antibody. In some species it may act to agglutinate small complexes of antigen, antibody, and complement, and promote their phagocytosis.

13.2 ACQUIRED IMMUNITY

It is worth reiterating that innate immunity may fail to provide defense against new and "unexpected" antigenic varieties of invading organisms. For this kind of rapid adaptation, vertebrates need their true immune system with its specific T cells and antibodies, produced, according to many immunologists, in almost endless diversity and by random processes. Here we will summarize the mechanisms known to be involved in acquired resistance to infectious disease before discussing those particularly relevant to various classes of parasite.

13.2.1 Antibody

The following four effects can be distinguished.

13.2.1.1 *Neutralization of toxins*

Combination near the active site of a toxin may stereochemically block its toxic activity. At a distant site, antibody may produce allosteric changes which inactivate the toxin. Toxin–antitoxin complexes are liable to phagocytosis.

13.2.1.2 *Lysis*

In the presence of complement, IgM and IgG antibodies may lyse bacteria, particularly gram-negative organisms, as discussed earlier. Some virus-infected cells are also lysed in this way.

13.2.1.3 *Recruitment of phagocytic cells*

Apart from their increased susceptibility to phagocytosis, antibody–bacteria complexes activate the complement system producing local inflammatory and chemotactic effects.

13.2.1.4 *Virus neutralization*

Antibody limits the spread and multiplication of many viruses by promoting their phagocytosis, and preventing their attachment to susceptible cells. Viruses with envelopes may be lysed by antibody plus complement. IgA antibody at mucous surfaces helps prevent access of viruses and bacteria by some mechanism which is not yet understood.

13.2.2 Cell-Mediated Immunity

Historically there has been an unwarranted preoccupation with antibody alone as the effector of immune resistance. It is easy to obtain immune serum and, after transferring it to a normal individual, to look for passively acquired immunity. However, in the early years of this century it became evident that in certain diseases like tuberculosis, antibody was not protective. In 1921, Zinsser found that a state of immunity to tuberculosis was accompanied by delayed-type hypersensitivity (Section 9.4.2). In 1942, Chase and Landsteiner showed that this immunity could be transferred to normal animals with lymphoid cells, but not with serum. Hence the term "cell-mediated immunity" (CMI). It is not an ideal name; after all, antibody is also produced by cells. However, the expression is now applied to those immunological mechanisms mediated by T cells, with or without macrophage participation, which do not involve B cells.

As discussed in Section 9.4, we can distinguish two categories of "CMI T cells": (1) those with direct complement-independent cytotoxic effects on other (target) cells such as allografts or virus-infected cells; and (2) those which, on contact with antigen, liberate lymphokines (Section 9.4.3) that have a variety of effects on other cells. This second type of cell is responsible for the local inflammation, elicited by antigen in delayed-type hypersensitivity. It is also the prime mover in the phenomenon of "macrophage activation," very important in resistance to some infections. Immunity to bacteria which multiply in normal macrophages—*Mycobacterium, Brucella, Salmonella, Listeria*—depends heavily on the increased phagocytic and bactericidal power displayed by lymphokine-activated macrophages. Resistance to some protozoan and metazoan parasites is also mediated by activated macrophages. It will be recalled from Chapter 9 that this kind of CMI reaction has two stages: the first is a *specific* combination of antigen and T cell, and the second, a variety of nonspecific effects such as recruitment of phagocytes, activation of macrophages, and blastogenesis of local lymphocytes. Cell-mediated immunity seems generally to be more important than antibody in defense against agents which multiply inside cells, such as viruses, some protozoa, and bacteria.

13.2.3 Antibody and Cells Together

Antibody and nonspecific effector cells can often work together to destroy or remove foreign cells and particles. Two mechanisms may be distinguished, both depending on the fact that the effector cell has receptors for the Fc part of IgG and sometimes for C3, a component of complement (Fig. 13.2).

13.2.3.1 *Opsonization, followed by phagocytosis*

The uptake of molecular or small particulate antigens after coating with IgG antibody depends on an initial combination with Fc receptors on the plasma

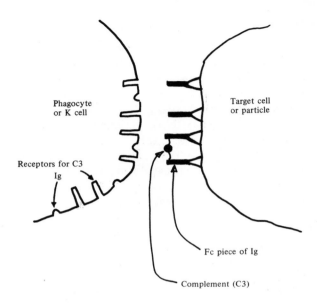

Fig. 13.2 Attachment of phagocyte or K cell to "target" particle coated with antibody, with or without complement.

membrane of the granulocyte or macrophage. Bound components of complement may assist the attchment through other receptor sites (Fig. 13.2). Phagocytic engulfment follows. (While phagocytes do not have receptors for the Fc piece of IgM antibody, they may, via their complement receptors, take up particles to which IgM antibody and complement are bound.)

13.2.3.2 *Antibody-dependent cell-mediated cytotoxicity (K cell killing)*

A class of small mononuclear cells known as K cells can also attach to the Fc part of IgG bound to target cells. There is disagreement as to whether complement may assist this union. In any case, these cells, after attachment to this cell-bound antibody, can directly destroy target cells which may be tumors, allografts, or cells infected with protozoa or microorganisms.

One might ask: "Why doesn't serum Ig inhibit this useful Fc-mediated binding of immune complexes to phagocyte and K cell surfaces?" Such inhibition can be shown *in vitro,* but it may be that *in vivo* the *multipoint* binding between an array of Fc pieces, perhaps together with complement, and their corresponding array of receptors is too strong to be inhibited by competition from monovalent Fc pieces on free IgG (Fig. 13.2). It is also possible experimentally to produce "armed macrophages," pretreated with cytophilic Fc-attached antibody molecules, which will then bind antigen via their Fab combining sites. However, it seems unlikely that such cells are important in the body since if single Fc combinations with their receptors were normally stable, all macrophages would be saturated with a heterogeneous array of irrelevant IgG molecules.

13.3 THE IMMUNE RESPONSE TO DIFFERENT CLASSES OF INVADING ORGANISMS

Two major points should emerge from this section. First, there is a surprising lack of precise knowledge about the immune mechanisms operating against many common infectious organisms, particularly protozoa and helminths. This is partly due to the complexity of responses to living invaders and the difficulty of determining which aspects of these responses are important, and partly to the difficulty of finding experimental models which accurately represent those diseases of humans and domestic animals with which we are ultimately concerned. Second, the immune response is not always very effective. Parasitic organisms have evolved various strategies of defense against the host immune response. The small, rapidly multiplying bacteria and viruses often pass on to new hosts before the original patient has had time to destroy them with an immune response. Many viruses and protozoa prolong their survival by generating new antigenic variants as antibodies to the original types arise. By contrast the larger, slower-breeding helminths often rely on "looking" antigenically as much like their hosts as possible so as not to induce a strong immune response, or simply on being hardy enough to weather the immunological storm which they provoke. In this section we will briefly examine the kinds of immune reaction stimulated by viruses, bacteria, protozoa, and some helminths.

13.3.1 Viruses

An important first line of defense against virus infection is provided by the fixed tissue macrophages, notably the alveolar macrophages which phagocytize airborne viruses, and the phagocytic cells lining the small blood vessels of liver, bone marrow, and spleen, which dispose of particles from the blood. There is a correlation between the virulence of viruses and their ability to multiply in macrophages; for example, newborn animals are often more susceptible to virus disease than adults, and their macrophages have low virucidal powers. Antibody greatly enhances phagocytosis and thus clearance of virus from the body.

The increased susceptibility of thymus-deficient humans and of T cell-depleted (e.g., thymectomized) animals to viral infection shows that CMI is vital in recovery from primary infection, particularly against those agents like poxviruses, herpesviruses, and measles virus, which pass directly from cell to cell. It is thought that CMI reactions protect the host in two ways: first, by destroying infected cells with cytotoxic T lymphocytes, and second, by the liberation, from sensitized T cells, of lymphokines which recruit and activate macrophages at the site of infection. A characteristic feature of many virus infections is their short incubation period, and part of the predominant importance of T cells in resistance to such infections may be attributed to the fact that the CMI response is quicker than antibody production. Interferon, produced even more rapidly, is also important. However, circulating antibody is very useful in preventing reinfection by many viruses, and in decreasing the spread of arboviruses and enteroviruses (e.g., hypogammaglobulinemics are more liable than normal to paralytic poliomyelitis). IgA at seromucous surfaces diminishes access of viruses, e.g., influenza, rhinoviruses, and coronaviruses (the last two being agents of the common cold) in respiratory passages.

While some viruses (measles, mumps, rubella, chickenpox, and smallpox) do not often undergo antigenic variation, and rely on a supply of new, nonimmune hosts for their continued propagation, others exist in a variety of antigenic forms, e.g., influenza, dengue, and poliovirus. Influenza produces recurrent human pandemics, each caused by radically new antigenic variants which emerge every few years. The disease is immunologically interesting since immunity to an older strain not only fails to protect an individual against new variants, but may even be actively harmful! This is because of the phenomenon known as "original antigenic sin." First contact with an initial or older strain, O, induces anti-O antibodies. Contact with a new strain, N, which would give anti-N antibodies in a person not previously infected with influenza, stimulates more anti-O antibodies in the O-immune individual. These antibodies are not protective against N. The mechanism is probably as described in Fig. 13.3. Because immune induction is degenerate (Chapter 11), anti-O memory cells can be induced by virus N to make anti-O antibodies. By some regulatory effect, not yet understood, this vigorous anti-O response may rapidly induce a compensating suppression which at the same time prevents the specific anti-N primary response from producing protective levels of antibody.

Another viral strategy for avoiding immune reactions is the "vertical transmission" of infectious particles from mother to offspring, the viral antigens reaching the offspring early enough to induce tolerance rather than immunity. Transmission may be via placenta, milk, the cytoplasm of the fertilized egg, or even in a DNA copy of the viral genome integrated into host chromosomes, as with some animal tumor viruses (Chapter 14). An example of a vertically transmitted virus whose study has greatly influenced immunological ideas is the agent of lymphocytic choriomeningitis in mice. This produces disease when mice are first infected as adults, but when vertically transmitted, leads to a lifelong, inapparent infection. Viral antigen is abundant, and indeed transfer of normal lymphoid cells to an infected host may provoke an immune response which is harmful to

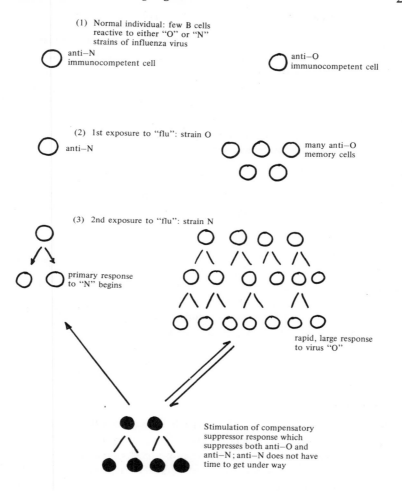

Fig. 13.3 Original antigenic sin: possible explanation.

the host. Yet the mice are essentially tolerant of the virus: they seem to regard it as part of self. This observation was one which contributed to Burnet and Fenner's early formulation of the concept of immunological tolerance.

13.3.2 Bacteria

The acquired mechanisms responsible for antibacterial immunity have been covered in Section 13.2. Antibody is thought to be particularly important in infections caused by *Streptococcus*, *Pneumococcus*, *Meningococcus*,

Pseudomonas aeruginosa, and *Haemophilus influenzae.* Antibody neutralizes toxins, and lyses some organisms if complement is available. When combined with particulate antigen, such antibody binds complement, induces local macrophage activation, and promotes phagocytosis. The existence of cell-mediated immunity may be inferred when specific skin tests of infected individuals show delayed-type hypersensitivity, as occurs in tuberculosis, brucellosis, typhoid (carrier state), syphilis, leprosy, melioidosis, and lymphogranuloma venereum. Such skin sensitivity presumably indicates that similar local reactions are occurring at foci of infection elsewhere in the body. However, it does not necessarily mean that CMI is essential for effective immunity: e.g., in *Staphylococcus aureus* and *Streptococcus pyogenes* infections, delayed hypersensitivity can be demonstrated, yet antibody confers immunity. We have already discussed the ability of some bacteria to multiply inside phagocytes, and the importance of the following pathway:

Sensitized T cell + antigen → lymphokines → macrophage activation →
                                                    increased nonspecific phagocytosis and killing.

Where the parasite is sufficiently hardy to resist killing even by activated macrophages, as are many mycobacteria, chronic local antigenic stimulation may occur, encouraging the formation of granulomata. These are collections of inflammatory cells in which macrophages predominate. Their presence may have pathological consequences, but they may also serve to "wall off" the focus of infection and diminish further spread of the organism.

13.3.3 Protozoa

The pathogenic protozoa and metazoa can often successfully parasitize a single host for long periods: naturally developing immunity is obviously not very effective in these cases. This is not to deny that protective vaccines might eventually be produced (as has been done for such persistent microorganism-induced diseases as tuberculosis), but it is difficult to establish that any immune response accompanying such natural infection has clinical relevance. As a rough generalization, humoral immunity is said to be significant against protozoa in the blood, while CMI is more important against parasites in tissues. Among the mechanisms which help these organisms to resist the host immune response are: their complex life cycles, often involving many antigenically different stages; their intracellular location in many cases; possibly some release of "blocking" antigens (and see Section 14.3.4 for discussion of this effect in the resistance of tumors to immune attack); sometimes the acquisition of a "coat" of host antigens; immunosuppression of the host by the parasite in some instances. Trypanosomes and malaria organisms may also undergo repeated antigenic changes within infected hosts. These appear to be alterations in phenotypic expression of antigen rather than selection of genetic variants, and are induced by antibody in the host, implying that immune responses against these parasites are sufficiently effective to have forced them to evolve this interesting mechanism for evading rejection.

The most important protozoan diseases of man are leishmaniasis, trypanosomiasis, and malaria. Malaria alone causes some one hundred million cases per year in tropical Africa, with a million deaths. The disease induces increased antibody formation whose clinical importance is uncertain. A beneficial increased cellular resistance is manifested by more rapid clearing of parasites and infected erythrocytes from the blood of immune people. Some resistance is transferable by cells or hyperimmune serum in experimental *Plasmodium* (malaria) infections of rats and mice. *Leishmania tropica* causes oriental sore, a disease which is accompanied by strong delayed-type hypersensitivity. In *L. donovani* infections (Kala azar) the situation is similar to malarial infections, with considerable antibody formation of unknown significance. In trypanosomiasis, evidence for useful overall protective immunity is still weak, although people and cattle in endemic areas are said to be relatively resistant to the disease.

13.3.4 Helminths

The most important helminth diseases in man are schistosomiasis and hookworm infestation. *Schistosoma* species, which are responsible for an estimated one hundred million infections in humans, are trematodes living especially in mesenteric veins. The adults acquire host antigens in their outer coats which protect them against attack, but host immune reactions are known to occur, and although the adults persist, the immature migratory schistosomula may be destroyed. CMI is thought to be more important than antibody in this resistance to reinfection. Allergic reactions to antigens of the parasite eggs contribute to the disease. There are intriguing recent reports that schistosomula may be destroyed *in vitro* by the combined action of immune serum (without complement) and eosinophils.

Hookworms are gut-dwelling, blood-sucking nematodes. They stimulate a range of immune responses, which may result in expulsion of adult worms, in a reaction which appears to involve both antibody and sensitized lymphocytes. Helminths also characteristically induce elevated levels of IgE antibody, eosinophils, and mast cells in the blood, which has led to the suggestion that local anaphylactic reactions (Section 12.2.3), with release of vasoactive amines, may contribute to the expulsion of worms.

13.4 IMMUNOLOGICAL INTERVENTION

In human and veterinary medicine, infectious diseases can be controlled in three main ways: (1) by improving hygiene, e.g., good sanitation, improved cooking methods, destroying the mosquito vectors of malaria, wearing boots in areas where schistosome larvae would otherwise enter through the skin of exposed feet; (2) by treating established infections with drugs, such as antibiotics. Although these two modes of controlling infectious diseases are immensely important, they do have some disadvantages: hygienic improvements are not always economically feasible; drugs can only be given after infection is clinically obvious, by which time the patient may have suffered some damage; many chemotherapeutic agents have harmful side effects, which reflects the difficulty of interfering with the parasite's metabolism without harming that of the host; effective drugs are not yet available for all diseases. (3) The third method is by immunological manipulations which include (a) immunological diagnosis of present or past infection, such as testing serum antibody titers; (b) vaccination, with the aim of inducing immunity to natural infection without having to experience the actual disease; (c) immunological treatments, restricted mainly at present to administering immune antisera to, for example, suspected cases of tetanus infection.

13.4.1 Diagnostic Tests

Serum antibody tests are the simplest way of detecting prior exposure to a wide variety of infectious organisms. A rising titer with time indicates recent infection.

The most important diagnostic indication of a state of cell-mediated immunity is the skin test for delayed-type hypersensitivity. In humans there are a variety of such specific tests available, e.g., injection of mumps antigen, used to test for CMI to mumps virus, "brucellin" for brucellosis, "histoplasmin" for histoplasmosis, and a purified protein derivative of *Mycobacterium tuberculosis* for tuberculosis. *In vitro* tests on isolated lymphocytes are being increasingly explored as indicators of CMI, e.g., sensitized lymphocytes may transform into blast cells and divide when exposed to specific antigen; the normal migration of macrophages from a capillary tube is inhibited by the reaction between antigen and sensitized lymphocytes. Better standardization of CMI tests is needed. It would also be extremely helpful to have a single-cell test, analogous to the hemolytic plaque assay for antibody forming cells, for detecting sensitized T lymphocytes.

13.4.2 Vaccination

The objective of vaccination is to induce immunity in a form which prevents natural infection, and to do this without harming the patient. We have already discussed, in Chapter 2, how Jenner converted folklore into scientific fact with his investigations on the immunity to smallpox conferred by deliberate inoculation of people with cowpox. We saw also how Pasteur generalized this principle: virulent organisms could be attenuated, converted into less dangerous but still immunogenic forms, by a variety of procedures including simple aging of a culture (chicken cholera bacillus), gentle heating (anthrax bacillus), or serial passage through an unusual host species (rabies). Today, a variety of attenuated viral and bacterial vaccines are in common use (Table 13.2).

In 1886, Salmon and Smith made the important discovery (with chicken cholera) that killed organisms could also provoke useful immunity. Killed vaccines are now also widely available (Table 13.2). Living vaccines usually induce better immunity than killed material, presumably because the dead organisms do not reach the same parts of the body in the same amounts as natural infectious agents. For very prolonged immunity, antigen may need to persist (Chapter 6), and the retention of small numbers of virions may underlie the common long-lasting immunity to viruses (lifelong in the case of yellow fever, for example).

To counteract the harmful effects of invading organisms it is sometimes sufficient to immunize against their toxic products (Table 13.3). In 1923, Glenny and Ramon independently discovered that mild formaldehyde treatment of diphtheria toxin could destroy its toxic activity without affecting its antigenicity. Toxin was converted into "toxoid." Tetanus toxoid was also made and first widely used in World War II when it virtually abolished tetanus infection of wounds. Today, public health immunization programs have almost eliminated a number of diseases such as polio, diphtheria, and smallpox from many communities.

TABLE 13.2
Examples of Human Vaccines

Class of vaccine	Living	Dead
Toxoids		Diphtheria Tetanus
Bacteria	BCG (=Bacillus Calmette Guerin, against tuberculosis)	Cholera Pertussis Plague Typhoid
Viruses	Measles Mumps Polio (Sabin) Smallpox Yellow fever Rubella	Influenza Rabies Polio (Salk)
Rickettsia		Typhus Rocky Mountain spotted fever

TABLE 13.3
States of Acquired Immunity

State of immunity	How acquired
Active	Natural
	Recovery from infection
	Induced
	Dead vaccines
	Toxoids
	Killed organisms
	Living attenuated organisms
Passive	Natural
	Maternal antibody
	Induced
	Artificially transferred antibody

13.4.3 Immunological Treatments

By contrast with the preventive aspirations of vaccination, treatments aim to improve the lot of patients already infected. The most common current procedure is the transfer of passive immunity with antiserum. Antibody to tetanus, diphtheria, and botulinus toxins are commonly used, human material being preferable to antisera from horses or other species because of the danger of serum sickness when large amounts or repeated doses of foreign proteins are administered (Section 12.2.4). Human gamma globulin is sometimes given to people in contact with hepatitis, smallpox, or measles. To the newborn mammal, its mother is an important natural source of passive immunity (Table 13.3), antibody being absorbed from colostrum, via the intestine of the suckling youngster, and, in some species, across the placenta.

Active immunization of infected individuals is too slow to be helpful against most viral and bacterial infections, except for rabies where this kind of treatment has been practised since Pasteur's time. The transfer of sensitized lymphoid cells instead of serum is limited by the inevitability of their rejection within weeks; as we saw in Section 10.8, antigens on lymphocytes of other members of the same species are much more immunogenic than antigens on their serum proteins. Lymphocyte transfer has, however, been used to treat chronic candidiasis and vaccinia gangrenosa. To combat broader immunodeficiencies, thymus-deficient children have received thymus transplants, and stem cell-deficient patients, bone marrow, although in this latter case graft versus host disease may cause complications (Section 10.6). "Transfer factor" is a low molecular weight, nucleic acid-containing extract of human lymphocytes which has recently been used to transfer therapeutically useful levels of cell-mediated immunity to patients with certain fungus diseases, such as candidiasis. Its mode and specificity of action are still uncertain.

13.4.4 Possible Future Developments

Many existing vaccines could be improved. For living preparations there is often a small but real risk of reversion to virulence or of complications, such as encephalitis, which may outweigh the benefits of vaccination once the probability of contracting the natural disease is very low. There are also many important diseases against which vaccines are still either not available or not fully effective. In some of these, it seems that cell-mediated immunity would provide best protection, e.g., typhoid, leprosy, syphilis, and many diseases caused by protozoa and metazoa. In other instances, the mechanism of naturally acquired immunity is uncertain: trachoma, typhus, dengue, tick-borne encephalitis, hepatitis A and B, and chronic gonorrhea. In developing a new vaccine it is important, first of all, to seek evidence that immune resistance can be acquired. The relative importance of CMI and antibody formation should then be evaluated, and a convenient source of antigen sought which will induce immunity of the most effective kind. The site at which immunity is provoked is also often critical, for example, resistance to influenza may depend largely on IgA levels in the respiratory tract. Ideally, one wants to study "model" infection in experimental animals which mimic the natural disease of humans or domestic animals.

Vaccines are badly needed for many protozoan and helminth diseases. Three helminth vaccines are currently used, all in veterinary practice, against *Dictyocaulus viviparus* in cattle, *D. filaria* in sheep, and *Ancylostoma caninum* in dogs. All of these vaccines are irradiated immature forms of the worms. The problems of developing vaccines against well-adapted, antigenically varying organisms are immense, but it is vital that current efforts be continued and expanded because of the enormous numbers of people affected by many of these diseases.

For treatments, as opposed to vaccination, the aim is to amplify an existing immune response, or to change its character, usually from an antibody to a CMI response. Advances in chemotherapy have removed the need for immunological treatment of most bacterial diseases, and viral infections often progress too rapidly for immune intervantion to be worthwhile, but there seems to be considerable scope for immunology in many chronic protozoan, metazoan, and fungus-induced diseases, as well as in some chronic bacterial and viral infections such as leprosy and herpes. Various empirical measures can be attempted, such as injecting extracts of mycobacteria to stimulate nonspecific local immunity. This has apparently been shown to induce some resistance to *Babesia* and *Plas-*

modium, and has also been used in tumor therapy (Section 14.5). Antigenic extracts of infectious organisms can be made and tested in experimental models. However, a rational approach would seem to depend, as in so much of immunology, on a better knowledge of immune *control.* We need to know how to control the amount, the class, and the specificity of immune responses: the amount, so as to boost inadequate reactions to useful levels (and this may involve circumventing suppressor reactions); the class, so as to promote CMI rather than antibody where needed, and vice versa; and the specificity, so as to divert responses away from older variants of such organisms as influenza and the trypanosomes which rely on remaining one antigenic jump ahead of an insufficiently changeable immune response.

13.5 SUMMARY

1. Vertebrates have evolved nonspecific innate mechanisms to protect themselves against parasites. These include humoral substances and phagocytic cells.

2. Most parasites, especially microorganisms, can multiply much more rapidly than their hosts, and generate new variants against which the host species has no effective innate defense.

3. The immune response is a mechanism evolved by vertebrates to allow rapid reaction against new parasites, antigenically distinct from self.

4. Among immune resistance mechanisms are: specific antibody, cell-mediated immune responses initiated by T cells, activation of macrophages, combined effects of antibody with phagocytes or K cells.

5. Parasites have a variety of properties which help them to evade immune attack. These include:

(a) rapid transmission to new hosts (notably viruses and bacteria)

(b) intracellular multiplication and resistance to phagocytic destruction (viruses, some bacteria, and protozoa)

(c) rapid antigenic variation of parasites within one host, ahead of the immune response (trypanosomes and malaria)

(d) immunosuppression of the host (e.g., trypanosomes and malaria)

(e) periodic antigenic variation, coupled with a tendency of the host to give an ineffective secondary response against the old strain of the organism (influenza)

(f) incorporation of host antigens into the outer coat of the parasite (some protozoa and helminths)

(g) resistance to immune mechanisms (e.g., some helminths, mycobacteria)

6. Knowledge of immune mechanisms against many organisms, particu-

larly protozoa and helminths, is still very imprecise. Among the reasons for this are the following:

(a) The parasites are complex organisms, often having many different forms during their life cycle, some of which may exist outside the vertebrate host.

(b) There are often no diseases in experimental animals which mimic the diseases of importance to humans, making them difficult to study.

(c) Immune responses are often themselves complex, and it is difficult to know exactly what is happening and what facets of the responses are important.

FURTHER READING

13.1   Burnet, F. M. and White. D. O. (1972). "Natural History of Infectious Disease," 4th ed. Cambridge Univ. Press, London.

13.2   Moller, G. (ed.). (1974). Immune Response to infectious diseases. *Transplant. Rev.* **19.** A collection of papers on this topic.

13.3   Nelson, D. S. (ed.). (1976). "Immunobiology of the Macrophage." Academic Press, New York.

13.4   Notkins, A. L. (ed.). (1975). "Viral Immunology and Immunopathology." Academic Press, New York.

13.5   Ogilvie, B. M. and Jones, V. E. (1973). Immunity in the parasitic relationship between helminths and hosts. *Prog. Allergy* **17,** 94.

13.6   "Cell-mediated immunity and resistance to infection." (1973). *W.H.O. Tech. Rep. Ser.,* Geneva.

QUESTIONS

13.1   An animal is immunized with two unrelated kinds of bacteria, *Salmonella* and *Streptococcus*. When some of its macrophages are removed, washed, and examined *in vitro*, these cells very efficiently phagocytize either kind of bacteria, even in the absence of any immune serum. A friend of yours says this shows that macrophages do not depend on Ig opsonins for phagocytosis. You maintain that the cells have cytophilic antibody, but, to your embarrassment, this cannot be directly demonstrated by fluorescence-labeled anti-Ig staining. Devise a simple experiment to prove that these macrophages do require some kind of specific immune recognition for efficient phagocytosis of the bacteria.

13.2   As the veterinarian in a small country district you wish to confirm a suspicion, based on clinical examination, that a herd of cattle has recently been exposed to *Brucells abortus* infections, and that the infection is slowly spreading through the herd. What confirmation might you seek?

13.3   Why are people who have recovered from an attack of one strain of influenza virus sometimes less able than previously unaffected individuals to resist infection by a new strain of influenza?

14

Cancer Immunology

During normal development cells proliferate to form tissues. This growth is strictly regulated: cell multiplication stops when an organ reaches its normal full size. Cancer, an aberration of this process, is the group of diseases resulting when a cell and its descendants undergo some change which allows them to escape from these controls and to proliferate in an abnormal and harmful way. Almost any of the tissues in the body may be affected, producing a great variety of syndromes. Cancer is, of course, a major cause of human death. Existing treatments are still relatively crude: surgical removal of lesions before they have had a chance to spread; local irradiation of tumors; mitotic poisons which selectively destroy rapidly dividing cancer cells. No really rational immunotherapy exists, yet, as we shall see, there is evidence that immune responses against cancer cells do occur, and although these responses are often ineffective, there is reason to hope that they can be artificially improved. Cancer immunology warrants a separate chapter because it is a fascinating biological problem, because it is important in human clinical medicine, and, above all, because a better understanding of basic immunology may eventually lead to cures for at least some cancers.

A "tumor" is, strictly speaking, any abnormal swelling, but the word is commonly used to mean a local cancerous growth. A "neoplasm" (lit. "new growth") is a more precise term for the same thing. Cancers may be benign or malignant. Benign neoplasms usually involve relatively differentiated cells and are slow growing and localized. Malignant growths, which are much more dangerous, are characterized by fast development, invasion of local tissue, and dissemination of neoplastic cells to other parts of the body (metastases). The cells in a neoplasm often bear little resemblance to their normal counterparts in the tissue from which they have arisen, and may rapidly change ("progress") with successive generations to variable and grossly abnormal forms.

216

14.1 DEVELOPMENT OF A TUMOR

Most neoplasms probably develop following an initial change in a single cell. Many neoplasms are known to be single clones, for example, the homogeneous myeloma proteins discussed in Chapter 3 come from malignant clones of antibody forming cells. This cancerous change is inherited by descendants of the original cell; it involves either an alteration in the DNA (produced, for example, by mutation or by integration of DNA from an "oncogenic" virus), or a stable change in the pattern of genes expressed by the DNA. As the tumor grows, further new genetic variants may appear which have increased proliferative power and so outgrow their neighbors. Advanced tumors commonly have a completely abnormal complement of chromosomes.

14.2 WHAT PROVOKES CANCER?

The inevitable question "What causes cancer?" gets us immediately into difficulties. For most diseases it is relatively easy to pinpoint a single cause: e.g., *Clostridium tetani* causes tetanus. Cancers, on the other hand, are almost certainly induced by combinations of events. Various agents, for example carcinogenic chemicals, ionizing radiation, or integration of viral nucleic acid into the genome, may produce changes in a cell which endow it with the potential to proliferate faster than its neighbors. Such changes may even occur spontaneously (i.e., without known cause), in rare cells. In many, perhaps most, cases, these altered cells are never noticed, because they are effectively controlled, by normal regulatory mechanisms. These controls are not well understood, but may include the tissue-specific antimitotic agents, "chalones," and probably systemic hormonal agents as well. Immune reactions may also eliminate some incipient neoplasms (see below).

The eventual emergence of a tumor probably follows the action of several chance events on the same cell. A second genetic change in a cell which has already mutated once may now render it less susceptible to regulation. A favorable environment for "escape" of the cell and its progeny may be provided by chronic local inflammation. The exponential increase in incidence of most cancers with age implies that more than one change is often needed to make a cell neoplastic. There is frequently a latency period, sometimes lasting many years, between application of a carcinogen and development of a tumor. Genetic factors in the host may also be important: certain human families and races develop some kinds of cancer with greater than average frequency; inbred strains of mice exist which have been selected for their high tumor incidence. Some viruses produce cancers in animals, and other have been associated with human neoplasms, but the significance of viruses in most human cancer is still uncertain. At present they should be thought of as only one among a variety of agents which may increase the probability of neoplastic changes in cells.

14.3 IMMUNE CONTROL OF CANCER

Tumor cells usually have surface antigens which are not present on normal cells. Thus they should be susceptible to immune attack. Why are some tumors not destroyed? Opinions on this question form a spectrum between two extremes. At one pole are those who say that the immune system is largely irrelevant in cancer, neoplastic growths being normally checked by nonimmunological homeostatic mechanisms. At the other extreme is the immune surveillance theory discussed later in this chapter: the view that the major reason for evolution of an immune system in the first place was to combat cancer (and parasites), and that the great majority of neoplasms are destroyed by immune mechanisms before they reach noticeable size.

14.3.1 Immunogenicity of Tumors

Tumors can induce specific immunity. A classic type of experiment is shown in Fig. 14.1. Spontaneously arising or carcinogen-induced tumors, which may kill the original animal, will not usually "take" in another genetically different individual of the same species. However, such tumors can be freely transplanted between genetically identical (isogeneic) animals. (This kind of experiment was in fact important in the early development of transplantation theory.) Injection of irradiated cells from a tumor will often confer resistance to subsequent challenge with live cells. The immunity is specific: growth of an unrelated tumor is not affected. The antigens responsible for this immunity are called "tumor-specific transplantation antigens" (TSTA), or "tumor-associated rejection antigens." This potential immunity focuses attention on our basic practical problem: "Why didn't the original animal destroy its own tumor?"

Immunity may often be passively transferred to normal animals using lymphoid cells taken either from the first host or from immunized individuals (Fig. 14.1). Transferred serum is not usually protective except in the case of some tumors, like leukemias, whose cells are dispersed rather than growing in a solid mass. The protective effect of cells but not serum is reminiscent of experiments on the transfer of delayed hypersensitivity (Section 9.4.2; and see below).

14.3.2 Tumor Antigens

Tumors in different individuals caused by the same oncogenic (tumor-generating) virus have common antigens. This is hardly surprising since the viral

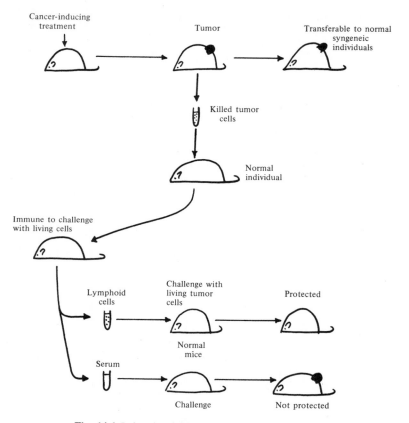

Fig. 14.1 Induced and adoptive immunity to neoplasms.

genome contributes to the changed pattern of surface components made by the neoplastic cells. Examples are murine sarcoma and polyoma viruses in mice, and fibroma virus in rabbits. Immunization with one tumor will confer resistance to challenge with another caused by the same virus. By contrast, tumors arising spontaneously or induced by carcinogenic agents (e.g., methylcholanthrene, benzopyrene) have individually specific antigens. The same agent acting, for example, on the skin on opposite sides of the same mouse, will induce tumors with distinct antigens.

Antigenic cross-reactions between different tumors sometimes occur, however. An interesting recently recognized group are the "oncofetal" antigens which may be expressed by different tumors of the same cell type and also by embryonic cells. It seems that when cells become neoplastic they often dedifferentiate and reactivate genes coding for surface components which were made earlier in the ontogeny of that cell type. Examples are α-fetoprotein, associated with hepatomas, and carcinoembryonic antigen, a human glycoprotein found preferentially in fetal and tumoral tissues of the digestive tract.

14.3.3 Immune Reactions Against Tumors

There are four main types (Fig. 14.2) of immune reactions against tumors.

14.3.3.1 *Antibody plus complement*

Cytotoxic antibodies may destroy some dispersed cell tumors and help to prevent metastasis of others, such as malignant melanoma. In many cases, how-

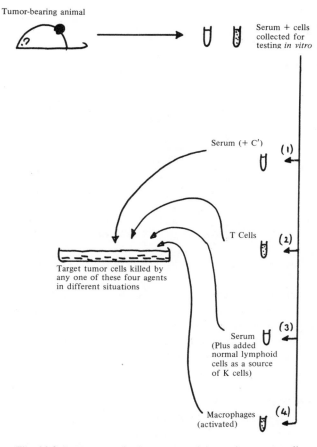

Fig. 14.2 *In vitro* tests for immune reactivity against tumor cells.

ever, antibody, far from being protective, may actually enhance tumor growth (see below).

14.3.3.2 *Activated specific T cells*

Cytotoxic cells with receptors specific for tumor antigens are an important means of killing neoplastic cells, particularly in the early stages of their growth. It seems likely that the other effector T cell pathway discussed in Section 9.4.3 may also be helpful: specific T cells are stimulated by tumor antigens to release lymphokines and provoke a local delayed-type hypersensitivity response. Macrophages are activated; nonspecific tissue damage occurs.

14.3.3.3 *Antibody-dependent cell-mediated cytotoxicity*

Until fairly recently, it was thought that "T cells are good and antibodies (because of their blocking activity) bad," in the immune response to most tumors. Now it seems that a cooperative effort by antibody and certain nonspecific lymphoid cells may damage tumors. The antibody must be of the IgG class. It combines with tumor antigens, leaving its Fc region exposed. Certain cells can attach to these Fc regions and thereby kill the tumor cell. Complement is not involved. Cells capable of this maneuver include macrophages and a class of lymphocytes called "K" cells which are certainly not T cells, and probably not B cells, i.e., they are a separate, small subclass of lymphocytes. In some instances, macrophages apparently become "armed" with cytophilic antibody before reacting against a tumor (cf. Section 13.2.3).

14.3.3.4 *"Activated macrophages"*

Normal macrophages will not kill tumor cells. However, they may become "activated" by exposure to lymphokines or to such substances as peptone broth, glycogen, or BCG (the tubercle bacillus vaccine strain). It seems that they will then kill neoplastic cells (there is still debate about this). It is difficult to see how this killing could be specific; probably normal cells in the vicinity are also killed.

Most of the evidence for the existence of these anti-tumor immune mechanisms comes from *in vitro* tests of serum and cells from tumor bearing animals or human patients (Fig. 14.2). It is extremely difficult to know how relevant these measurements are to *in vivo* immunity. For example, cytostatic effects (i.e., "cell-stopping" as opposed to cell killing) may be missed *in vitro* but vital in the body. In the other direction, *in vitro* assays may indicate good antibody dependent or cell-mediated killing of biopsied neoplastic cells while the tumor itself grows steadily. *In vivo* transfers of immune cells or serum between experimental animals give variable results. Yet immunosuppresive agents (drugs, antilymphocyte serum) will often increase the rate of growth of a tumor, suggesting that it was being at least hampered by immune mechanisms. The interesting phenomenon known as "concomitant immunity" also argues in favor of immune defense: an animal which is unable to halt the growth of its primary tumor will sometimes nevertheless reject cells from the same tumor which would have lodged and grown successfully in a normal individual. This may mean that metastases from the primary tumor are also destroyed. Excision of a primary malignant growth in human or experimental animals is sometimes followed by disappearance of remaining neoplastic cells. These are probably removed by immune mechanisms which were unable to cope with the more massive and inaccessible primary tumor.

14.3.4 Ways in Which Tumors Can Escape the Immune Response

A neoplasm should be thought of as a *population* of cells which behaves rather like a species of microorganism in an unfavorable environment. Many individuals fail to multiply at all. When one does begin to proliferate its descendents are continually seeking, as it were, to increase their chances of survival. Variants appear in the population, those with the greatest selective advantage having the fastest rates of proliferation, the least susceptibility to normal tissue growth controls, and usually the weakest immunogenicity. The more a tumor resembles "self" antigenically the less it is liable to rejection. Analogies may be drawn with metazoan parasites which sometimes surround themselves with host components to subvert immune attack, and with allografts which survive longest if they come from antigenically similar strains. There is an important difference however: grafts or parasites will die if a proportion of their cells are destroyed; a single tumor cell escaping death may kill the host.

Klein lists five reasons why tumors may escape immune destruction:

14.3.4.1 *Immunodeficiency of the host*

Tumor growth is often facilitated by immunosuppressive treatments, as mentioned earlier. In addition, individuals may be "genetically unresponsive" to some tumors as to other antigens (Section 11.3). For example, Gross virus in mice is vertically transmitted (from mother to offspring) and causes no tumors in most wild mice. An inbred strain, AKR, has been selected for susceptibility to tumor induction by the virus. The strain has a particular allele in the *H-2* region (Chapter 11) which determines this susceptibility.

14.3.4.2 *"Sneaking through"*

A tumor obviously presents a very small amount of new antigen to its host initially, and this increases steadily as the tumor proliferates. In some cases the amount of antigen may be too small to provoke a response until the tumor has already formed a clump of cells which is large enough to resist attack. Experimentally, the injection of a very small number of neoplastic cells may give a higher incidence of "takes" than administering a larger number. Cases are also known where injection of a relatively large number of irradiated tumor cells during the "latent" period of a tumor (i.e., when it is too small to be seen macroscopically) may prevent further growth and emergence of that tumor. The implication is that a sudden large dose of antigen jolts the immune system into action while the tumor is still small enough to be susceptible! Some intriguing recent experiments suggest that "sneaking through" is more than just a numbers game: a state of low zone tolerance (Section 6.9) to the tumor antigens may be induced during the early stages of the immune response which actively retards the subsequent immune reaction.

14.3.4.3 *Immunoresistance of tumors*

Tumors may develop a variety of properties which assist their survival. We have already discussed the concept that neoplasms evolve toward lower immunogenicity to avoid immune attack, and have touched on the obvious idea that the cells within a large, poorly organized lump may be relatively inaccessible to immune effector cells and antibodies. Some tumors secrete substances with antiinflammatory activities which prevent local mobilization of macrophages; some release factors which enhance blood vessel development and thus promote vascularization and growth of the tumor. There is a further very important trick displayed by some tumors which helps them to survive: antibody reacting with certain tumor antigens may "modulate" them, that is cause their disappearance from the cell surface. These cells then become insusceptible to attack by any immune mechanism directed against the modulated antigens. The ability to "shed" its surface antigens in this way seems to be correlated with tumor malignancy.

14.3.4.4 *Lack of recognition*

This refers again to the idea that weakly immunogenic tumors are difficult to reject.

14.3.4.5 *Malfunctioning of the immune system*

By this Klein means that a vigorous immune response may often be made, but prove ineffective. The blocking effect of antibody or antigen–antibody complexes is the most important example. As a tumor grows it "sheds" antigen. Thus the patient has, in his circulation, free antigen, free antibody, and antigen–antibody complexes, the proportion of each depending on the relative concentration of the reactants. Obviously, antigen has the potential to block receptors on cells capable of reacting against the tumor, while "enhancing" antibody has the power to cover surface antigens on neoplastic cells and shield them from immune attack by, for example, cytotoxic T cells. Such blocking effects can be shown by *in vitro* tests with serum from many tumor-bearing animals. It is now thought that the major blocking effect is caused by *complexes* of antibody with soluble tumor antigens, which explains why blocking activity often disappears when the tumor is excised (removing antigen) although free antibody levels may remain high.

14.3.5 Outline of Probable Events in an Immune Reaction to a Tumor

To summarize preceding sections we may consider the "life history" of a successful tumor. During its critical early phase of growth it will be subject to attack by cytotoxic T cells; there is some evidence that small amounts of antigen stimulate T cells more readily than B cells. Cytotoxic antibody is also most dangerous to the emerging neoplasms in its early stages. If it survives this onslaught, it grows and may shed significant amounts of antigen. More antibody is made at this stage; K cells provide a new line of host defense but antigen–antibody complexes often appear which block cellular attack. Most testing of patients is done at this stage. Finally, massive antigen release may block effector cells, and perhaps induce high zone tolerance. There is often general immunosuppression of the patient, and the tumor, having escaped all host control grows until its host succumbs.

14.4 THE IMMUNE SURVEILLANCE HYPOTHESIS

This is the view expressed by Thomas and developed by Burnet (Ref. 14.3) that the main evolutionary pressure for evolution and retention of an immune system has been to combat neoplasia. Burnet's reasoning is as follows. He believes that there is no true cancer among invertebrates (although other authors disagree). With the emergence of vertebrates came the risk, particularly among primitive cyclostome fish, that one individual would parasitize another of the same species. As a defense against this, two parallel mechanisms evolved. (1) There was a "loosening of somatic–genetic controls" to allow greater variation among somatic cells. This led to histocompatibility antigen polymorphism (Section 10.4.1) and had the desirable effect of making individuals within a species antigenically distinct. It also set the stage for neoplastic disease. (2) The immune system developed, primarily to react against neoplasms and intraspecies parasites.

Burnet proposes that there is rapid variation of histocompatibility antigens of normal somatic cells in vertebrates. The developing immune system is stimulated by these antigens, most of which are relatively similar in kind to the germline-inherited histocompatibility type. Thus there is a spontaneous priming against such antigens which is reflected in the high reactivity of lymphocytes to allogeneic cells (Section 10.10). The immune system becomes particularly efficient at eliminating incipient tumors, which look like allogeneic cells, and cancer is prevented from being a contagious disease because cells from one animal are rejected by another.

The great virtue of this theory is that it attempts to relate the two most highly polymorphic systems known: histocompatibility antigens and immunoglobulins. This theory is being increasingly criticized by immunologists, however. It is predicated on a high natural priming to alloantigens, and we have seen (Section 10.10) that there is probably no such immune preoccupation with alloantigens unless they are presented on lymphocytes. Furthermore, while immune responses can control certain tumors, they are not always very effective, as we have discussed. The most important prediction of the immune surveillance theory is that on removal of an individual's immune potential, neoplasms should increase significantly. The facts are as follows. Immunosuppression does greatly increase the susceptibility of animals to certain oncogenic viruses, but these experimental situations may not be relevant to spontaneous cancer in man. Congenitally immunodeficient children, and immunosuppressed patients (e.g., recipients of allografts) develop many more tumors than normal individuals, but these are nearly all lymphoid and reticular. According to the surveillance concept, all types of tumor should increase. Other possible explanations for the excessive *lymphoid* neoplasia are that the immunosuppressive drugs are themselves carcinogenic, or that suppressed individuals are subject to chronic antigen stimulation which they are unable to control. Nude mice and mice treated by thymectomy or antilymphocyte serum do not seem to show any spontaneously increased incidence of tumors, which is a damaging finding for immune surveillance. The theory cannot be rescued from this last observation by suggesting that these mice still have residual anti-tumor defenses, because the animals are greatly depressed in their ability to reject allografts, and graft and tumor rejection have been firmly tied together in the surveillance concept. It has even been suggested (by Prehn) that the immune system works to the advantage of tumors by mildly stimulating them!

A reasonable view at the moment would be that while the immune system helps to control tumors it is not nearly as efficient as we would like (Table 14.1 summarizes the arguments). This inefficiency is, however, a cause for optimism rather than despair, since it presents us with the challenge of improving the immune system's performance by manipulating it.

14.5 POSSIBLE IMMUNOTHERAPY AGAINST CANCER

A distinction should be made between prevention and treatment of cancer. Prevention depends on understanding causes and interfering with conditions that

TABLE 14.1
Evidence For and Against the Idea that the Immune System Plays an Important Role in Preventing Cancer[a]

For	Against
1. Most cancers have new antigens and provoke immune responses	Tumors are often weakly antigenic, and grow in spite of the immune response
2. Virus-induced (experimental) cancers may provoke good immunity	Such viral infections may not be an important cause of many natural cancers in humans
3. Some immune responses damage tumors. *In vitro,* cytotoxic T cells, antibody, and K cells can be demonstrated	Relevance of *in vitro* to *in vivo* reactions not clear. Some antibody responses protect tumors (antigen–antibody blocking complexes)
4. Greatly increased incidence of neoplasms in immunosuppressed individuals and congenitally immunodeficient children	These neoplasms are almost all lymphoreticular. Explanations other than decreased surveillance are possible
5. T cells can destroy tumors	"Nudity," and ALS treatment or thymectomy of mice does not increase the incidence of spontaneous neoplasms
6. Spontaneous cancers are not contagious	They are not contagious in inbred strains of animals
7. The immune system may destroy many more tumors than are ever seen	Precancerous and occult lesions may be common and persist without developing (implies nonimmune control?)
8. Vigorous immune response against allografts	Grafts cultured to remove lymphocytes may stimulate no rejection reaction

[a]Points (4–7) are especially relevant to the immune surveillance theory.

contribute to cancer. For example, carcinogenic chemicals can be identified, and sometimes eliminated from man's environment. Treatment, of course, applies to patients with an existing tumor. Most of our experience with cancer has been gained from study of the tumor bearing state, and it is worth reemphasizing that we still know very little about *natural resistance* and the extent to which immune mechanisms normally control the disease.

The point of immunological attack against a neoplasm must be those antigens in which it differs from the host. Most current cancer treatments are nonspecific (e.g., local irradiation, cytotoxic drugs) and damage cells other than the tumor: immunotherapy has the great potential advantage of affecting only those cells which bear the specific tumor antigens.

If it becomes established that viruses are an essential agent in the generation of some human cancers then antiviral vaccines can be considered. For spontaneous growths with unique antigens any "vaccine" would have to consist of an extract of that particular neoplasm. Tumor-specific antigens have been isolated, but not successfully used as therapeutic agents. Another approach has been to remove some neoplastic cells, modify them in some way *in vitro* to increase their immunogenicity (e.g., by infecting them with virus or coupling foreign antigens chemically), and then to inject these cells back into the original animal in the hope of stimulating a stronger or altered immune response against the tumor-specific antigens. This does not seem to have led to any consistent immunization schedules. A long-standing dream of cancer immunologists has been the "magic bullet" idea. Antibody against the tumor is made in normal individuals. This reagent should now, when injected, "home" specifically to the neoplastic cells (provided it has been suitably absorbed to remove antibodies against histocompatibility antigens). To this antibody various additional agents can be attached, e.g., highly radioactive compounds, or antimitotic drugs. The aim is to focus these substances directly on the tumor. So far this ingenious scheme has not yielded useful results.

The most hopeful kind of approach would seem to lie in better therapeutic control of the individual's own immune response to its cancer. For example, where antibodies are blocking a potentially useful cytotoxic T cell reaction, it should be possible to depress antibody production and encourage generation of more T cells, perhaps by decreasing the amount of tumor antigen available, or by removing some helper T cells from the animal. A currently popular clinical maneuver, injecting BCG (attenuated tubercle bacillus) plus irradiated tumor cells, may act by selectively stimulating cytotoxic T cells, or by activating macrophages. If antitumor responses are actively suppressed by lymphocytes, then removing suppressors may be beneficial. If self-tolerance is maintained by active suppression (Section 11.2.3), it is possible that immune responses to tumor antigens are often poor because of the strong suppression against self-components coupled to these tumor antigens: we may in the future learn how to "uncouple" the associated helper and suppressor effects of responses to linked antigens. In any case, rational treatments will depend on a vastly improved knowledge of immune control, which is perhaps the most practically important area of research in immunology at present.

14.6 SUMMARY

Cancer results from harmful overproliferation of cells. Some of the factors which contribute to this escape of cells from normal homeostatic controls are spontaneous mutation, oncogenic viruses, carcinogenic chemicals, irradiation, and favorable local tissue conditions for multiplication of abnormal cells. Immune responses can be made by animals against their tumors since these usually bear new antigens. The major immune mechanisms which may help to destroy tumors are cytotoxic T cells, cytotoxic antibodies, and cooperative effects between specific antibodies of IgG class and certain nonspecific lymphoid cells. Tumors often escape rejection, however, because they are antigenically weak, or inaccessible to immune effector cells. Antigen–antibody complexes may block the approach to a tumor of cells which might otherwise damage it. The immune surveillance theory and some possible immunotherapeutic approaches to cancer are briefly discussed.

FURTHER READING

14.1   Baker, M. A. and Taub, R. N. (1973). Immunotherapy of human cancer. *Prog. Allergy.* **17,** 227.

14.2   Becker, F. F. (1974). "Cancer: A Comprehensive Treatise," Vols. I–IV. Plenum, New York.

14.3   Burnet, F. M. (1970). "Immunological Surveillance." Pergamon Press, Oxford.

14.4   Burnet, F. M. (1973). Multiple polymorphism in relation to histocompatibility antigens. *Nature (London),* **245,** 359.

14.5   Hehlmann, R. (1976). RNA tumor viruses and human cancer. *Curr. Top. Microbiol. Immunol.* **73,** 141.

14.6   Hellstrom, K. E. and Hellstrom, I. (1974). Lymphocyte-mediated cytotoxicity and blocking serum activity to tumor antigens. *Adv. Immunol.* **18,** 209.

14.7   Mitchison, N. A. (1973). "Tumor immunology," *In* Essays in Fundamental Immunology" (I. Roitt, ed.). Vol. I, p. 44. Blackwell Scientific Publ., Oxford.

14.8   Moller, G. (ed.). (1976). Experiments and the concept of immunological surveillance. *Transplant. Rev.* **28.** A collection of papers criticizing the surveillance concept.

14.9   Nossal, G. J. V. (1974). "Lymphocyte differentiation and immune surveillance against cancer." *Develop. Aspects Carcinogenesis Immunity, 32nd Symp. Soc. Devel. Biol.,* p. 205. Academic Press, New York.

14.10 Smith R. T. and Landy, M. (eds.). (1974). "Immunobiology of the Tumor-Host Relationship." Academic Press, New York. Proceedings of a conference: very readable and stimulating.

14.11 Weiss, D. W. (1973). Immunological intervention in neoplasia. *In* "The Role of Immunological Factors in Viral and Oncogenic Processes" (R. F. Beers, R. D. Tilghman, and E. G. Bassett, eds.), p. 131. Miles Lab. 7th Int. Symp., Johns Hopkins Univ. Press, Baltimore, Maryland.

QUESTIONS

14.1   In Section 14.3.1 it was said that tumors induced in one strain of mice by a carcinogenic agent such as methylcholanthrene were rejected on transplantation to another strain of mice. Why? If treatment with a chemical carcinogen led to the formation of two separate solid tumors, how might you tell whether they were derived from the same or different initial neoplastic cells?

14.2   Why are "immune complexes" of tumor antigen plus antibody more efficient than free antigen at blocking anti-tumor-reactive cells? Why does excision of a primary tumor often remove such blocking activity from serum in spite of the fact that levels of antibody to the tumor remain high in the serum?

14.3   What are the main arguments for and against the immune surveillance theory? If it were demonstrated that all tumors are caused by extrinsic agents such as viruses, would this improve the evidence for the theory?

15

Evolution of the Immune System

Why do vertebrates have an immune system? The answer given in Chapter 1 was "for defense against infectious organisms." Then how do many invertebrates and plants manage without such a mechanism, since they are also liable to infectious disease? To understand any biological system, it is important to get some feeling for how and why it evolved. In this chapter we will briefly discuss why the development of an immune apparatus may have been essential for the evolution of more complex animals.

15.1 A RECAPITULATION OF THE PROPERTIES OF THE VERTEBRATE IMMUNE SYSTEM

We can see now how the basic requirements of an immune system (Chapter 1) have been met by vertebrates. Immune responses must be specific to avoid anti-self reactions: this specificity resides in the V regions of immunoglobulin antibodies, or in similar molecules on the surface of lymphoid cells. The great range of V region primary sequences ensures sufficient antibody diversity to cope with any antigen, but this diversity arises spontaneously within lymphocytes and is not fashioned around "instructive" antigen molecules. Antigen simply selects from the available repertoire. In the opinion of many immunologists it is the random nature of lymphocyte diversification that underlies the vertebrates' ability to react against unexpected antigens. Adaptivity is achieved by clonal selection: those lymphocytes to which antigen binds, proliferate, leaving behind a pool of memory cells ready to mediate a more rapid and vigorous secondary response. Perhaps the memory state involves also some disturbance of a regulatory equilibrium; it seems clear now that tolerance, the negative aspect of memory, is often caused by an increase in suppressor cell activity. The unique properties of the immune system are engineered by several unusual genetic mechanisms: translocation of V regions to different C region genes, allelic exclusion to facilitate selection of lymphocytes, and (probably) a high rate of somatic variation in V genes (Chapter 7).

15.2 PHYLOGENETIC EMERGENCE OF AN IMMUNE SYSTEM

15.2.1 Invertebrates

Invertebrates display "immunity" in that they often have macromolecules or cellular reactions which help to protect them against pathogenic microorganisms. Several invertebrate classes have been shown to have substances in their body fluids which can agglutinate foreign bacteria or other antigens, but while levels of these agglutinins are sometimes increased after injection of an antigen, the normal pattern is for constant amounts to be synthesized regardless of antigenic exposure, with no increase in titer on repeated challenge. The antigen binding molecules are diverse (different antigens do not absorb all of them) in some cases, but have very little specificity of action in others. In structure they seem to be very different from vertebrate antibody. Invertebrates often have "blind spots": pathogenic organisms and antigens against which they have no detectable reaction or defense.

Cellular reactions may be observed between members of different strains within certain invertebrate and plant species. For example, colonial tunicates fuse with genetically identical organisms, or with others which share one haplotype (Section 10.4.2), but refuse to unite with ("reject"?) colonies more genetically dissimilar. These reactions are not adaptive. Individuals do not learn from experience. Also, there are many instances among invertebrates where allografts and even tissues from different species are accepted as readily as autografts.

There is, however, some recent evidence for adaptive graft rejection among higher invertebrates, the annelids and echinoderms, which may herald the first phylogenetic emergence of true immune reactions. Annelids accept autografts but reject skin from other genera. The rejection is associated with an accumulation of coelomocytes around the graft. A second graft from the same donor is rejected more quickly and to the accompaniment of a more rapid congregation of coelomocytes. It would be extremely interesting to have information on the diversity of these coelomocytes; if they are acting like vertebrate lymphocytes they should show clonal differences. Attempts to induce specific tolerance in the higher invertebrates would also be valuable.

15.2.2 Vertebrates

Consistent signs of adaptive immunity, together with the first histological evidence of organized lymphoid tissue, appear in the lowest vertebrates, the cyclostomes. The lamprey has a rudimentary thymus and some lymphocytes. It accepts autografts, rejects allografts, and can be sensitized to tuberculin. It is, however, a very poor antibody producer. Once the true fishes are reached, we see a well-developed immune system, essentially of the mammalian kind. Both elasmobranch and teleost fishes produce antibody, although sharks make only one class of Ig which exists in both 19 S and 7 S forms. Bacterial antigens uniformly elicit agglutinating antibodies in fish, amphibians, birds, and reptiles, and specific memory can be shown. First- and second-set graft rejections (Section 10.3) are also demonstrable in all of these classes.

15.2.3 Self–Not Self Discrimination

It is important to recognize the fundamental distinction between immune and nonimmune recognition. All living things distinguish between different materials in their surroundings. *Amoeba* will accept some foods and reject others. Hemocytes in worms engulf invading bacteria, but not one another. In a perhaps analogous way, cells of the same kind will assort into homogeneous tissues in higher animals. This type of discrimination between self and foreign substances is a basic and essential property of living cells. It probably depends on some kind of limited library of receptor molecules inherited through the germline DNA. An individual *Amoeba,* for example, reacts in a predetermined way to a given set of stimuli. Adapting to a new stimulus requires an evolution of the whole species.

Contrast this with the vertebrate immune apparatus which is a highly specialized kind of recognition system designed to learn from its environment. It has to learn not to react against self (Section 8.2). It is vested in lymphocytes, and has various unique properties which we have already discussed. We should avoid a logical error which appears in some of the writing on the phylogeny of immunity—the assumption that anything which shows self–not self discrimination is in some sense an immune system. All cells distinguish self from not self to some extent. A vertebrate macrophage in the absence of antibody may take up foreign bacteria but not host red blood cells; here it is operating via its limited nonimmune recognition powers. In the presence of antibody it need only recognize as worthy of phagocytosis anything to which Ig has combined, thus relegating the self–not self decision to the immune system.

15.3 HOW DO MANY ORGANISMS MANAGE
WITHOUT AN IMMUNE SYSTEM?

To answer this question we should look for systematic differences between vertebrates, on the one hand, and the lower invertebrates, on the other. Such attempts are bound to be hampered by the existence of exceptional species of either kind. However, vertebrates have several broad properties which would seem to make an adaptive immune system much more vital to their survival. First, they generally live longer than invertebrates. Thus the individual has correspondingly more chance of encountering a pathogenic organism. With their long generation times, vertebrate species are much less able than invertebrates to counter, by genetic variation of their own, the rapid evolution of microorganism populations. Second, invertebrate species usually (not always) have many more members than vertebrate species. This allows death of the vast majority in any generation without jeopardizing the species. Those individuals which meet a pathogenic microorganism may simply die, unless they are themselves resistant variants. Most vertebrate species could not afford this kind of strategy.

A number of other reasons can be suggested for the development of an adaptive immune system by vertebrates, although it is difficult to know how important these rationalizations are. For example, vertebrates are usually highly complex, and are perhaps more liable to be incapacitated (prevented from reproducing) by even relatively slight structural damage inflicted by invading parasites (but complexity has its compensations: it allows an individual to support a "police force" of lymphocytes!). The increased adaptability brought about by vertebrate evolution, coupled with their longer life span, probably means that they encounter more variety of antigens in their environment than do most invertebrates; this may also have encouraged the development of an immune system.

15.4 COMPARISON OF THE STRATEGIES OF VERTEBRATES AND INVERTEBRATES

From our discussion of the logic of immunity (Chapters 1 and 8), its genetic basis (Chapter 7), and evolution (this chapter) we have reached a point from which we can at least partially resolve the central paradox of immunology: understanding how an individual acquires new characteristics by contact with its environment. It was this apparently unbiological behavior of the immune system which prompted the instructive theory of antibody synthesis (Section 7.1), a position from which the subject was rescued by Jerne and Burnet who realized that immune phenomena must be explained without violating Darwinian evolutionary principles.

Apart from brain functions, learning to adapt to unexpected changes in the environment is a property of populations, not of individuals. Microorganisms and invertebrate animals have genes coding for useful and protective macromolecules. When a new pathogen or harmful molecule, against which their inherited defenses are ineffective, appears in their environment, most members of the species may die, while a few variants form the basis of a new resistant

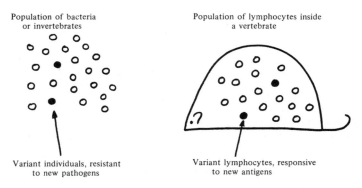

Population of bacteria
or invertebrates

Population of lymphocytes inside
a vertebrate

Variant individuals, resistant
to new pathogens

Variant lymphocytes, responsive
to new antigens

Fig. 15.1 Comparison of the immune strategies of vertebrates and invertebrates.

strain. Vertebrates have, however, a much more economical means of defense. They have developed an internal population of lymphocytes which behaves in many ways like an evolving species of invertebrates (Fig. 15.1). Variants appear in this population, and are selected by their antigenic environment. Lymphocytes "learn" in the same sense that a species learns, and their altered characters are passed on to their offspring. Their entire evolutionary history unfolds inside one "host." The host, by exploiting this population, can itself adapt to entirely new antigens, but using only classic evolutionary mechanisms. Vertebrate offspring do not inherit this acquired information but have to build up their own immunological repertoire.

These phylogenetic considerations are relevant to the old and still viable debate between germline and somatic theories of the genetics of antibody formation. There is no argument on how most properties of organisms evolve: random changes occur in the DNA and advantageous variants are selected. However, an individual cannot carry enough information in his DNA to anticipate all possible fluctuations of the environment. The same would seem to apply to lymphocytes.

15.5 SUMMARY

The first immune reactions—diverse, adaptive responses to entirely new antigens—appear phylogenetically with the higher invertebrates and lowest vertebrates. Most invertebrates appear to rely on conventional evolutionary strategy when faced with new, harmful antigens; many individuals die, and resistant variants are selected. Vertebrates have an additional mechanism, the immune system, which enables the *individual* to learn, during its own lifetime, to react against novel antigenic stimuli. An immune system is like a symbiotic population of unicellular organisms (lymphocytes) inside its vertebrate host. A great variety of different types (specificities) evolves within this population, some of them being encouraged by antigen to proliferate, secrete their specific products, and so provide protection for their host. Immune adaptation to entirely new antigens thus appears to depend ultimately on the classical evolutionary mechanism of individual (lymphocyte) variation and selection.

FURTHER READING

15.1 Cooper, E. L. (ed.). (1974). Invertebrate Immunology. *Contemp. Top. Immunobiol.* **4.** A large collection of articles on this topic, by different authors.

Appendix: Answers to Questions

CHAPTER 1

1.1 Immunosuppressant drugs are given to recipients of grafts to minimize their immunological reaction against foreign antigens of the graft, a reaction which usually causes graft rejection. Among the side effects are increased susceptibility to infections (Section 10.11.2).

1.2 The host would not now recognize the worm as foreign, and it would not provoke an immune reaction. Such means of defense are actually used by certain parasites (Sections 13.3.4).

1.3 The animal would have no reason to "see" the antigen as a foreign substance; it would instead be treated like a self-component. There would usually be no obvious immune reaction against such an antigen. This kind of situation has been created experimentally (Chapters 6, 8, 10; for complications, see Chapter 11).

1.4 Immunity to infectious diseases (including vaccination) (Chapter 13); graft rejection (Chapter 10); reactions against tumors (Chapter 14); autoimmune disease, allergies, and immune deficiencies (Chapter 12).

1.5 Species survive because of the random generation of genetic variants, some of which may be resistant to environmental changes which kill most members of the species. Among 10^{12} cells there must be many genetic variants, even assuming a "conventional" rate of variation, such as 10^{-9} variation events per base pair per generation. Variation in the cells of the immune system may be faster than this (with important implications for immunology, see Chapter 8).

CHAPTER 2

2.1 When mixed with the immunizing bacteria this antiserum agglutinated them, i.e., clumped them together. When dilutions of serum were tested, this agglutinating power was lost at dilutions greater than 1/10,000. Bacteria A were probably a closely related *Salmonella* species; B may have been less related (i.e., antigenically more different) *Salmonella* or possibly organisms of another genus; C was antigenically unrelated to *S. abortus-equi* according to the test used ("titers" of 1/2 are usually not considered significant since substances in serum other than specific antibody can give false agglutination reactions at low dilutions).

2.2 Antigen–antibody reactions are reversible, and complexes dissociate at a rate which depends on the affinity of the reaction (Section 2.3.3). Labeled antigen in such a complex would be slowly replaced by other (unlabeled) molecules, added later. That serum to which more unlabeled antigen needed to be added contained antibody with the higher affinity for antigen (assuming that both antisera were of the same class—Chapter 3).

2.3 When a relatively small amount of antigen (toxin) is added to a standard amount of antibody (antitoxin), this antigen may combine with more than its equivalent amount of antibody (zone of antibody excess, Fig. 2.5). There is now insufficient antibody left to neutralize completely the subsequently added toxin (within the time span of the experiment).

2.4 This would probably mean that the agglutinable red blood cells had, on their surfaces, antibody made by the individual against his own antigens. Such autoantibody is found in autoimmune hemolytic disease, and in some normal individuals. The antibody is said to be "incomplete" if it will not, by itself, agglutinate the red blood cells (Section 2.2.5); the reasons for such lack of agglutination are not completely clear.

If the rabbit antibody agglutinated erythrocytes from *any* human, we would be justified in suspecting that the serum contained anti-erythrocyte antibodies.

CHAPTER 3

3.1 A large proportion of the serum protein from the myeloma patient would be a single kind (amino acid sequence) of immunoglobulin made by a single clone, and therefore relatively homogeneous in its properties. Electrophoresis of the serum, for example, would produce a single very dense band superimposed on a normal pattern in case (b), as opposed to an overall increase in amount of globulins in (a).

3.2 By injecting labeled mouse IgG intravenously into another animal, and following rate of decay of label in subsequent daily bleeds. Radioactive tracers could be used, but perhaps the most elegant method would be to inject IgG antibody of high titer against a known antigen, and to measure the remaining titer in serum samples at intervals thereafter.

3.3 The IgM should bind more firmly (i.e., with greater *avidity*) since it combines with a valency of 5 (Section 3.2) as opposed to 2 for IgG.

CHAPTER 4

4.1 (a) A standard number of the spleen cells should produce about one-quarter as many plaques on goat as on sheep RBC, i.e., one-quarter of the antibody forming cells make antibody capable of lysing both kinds of erythrocyte. (b) On a mixed indicator layer (Section 4.6.2) we would see two kinds of plaque: 25% would be "clear," with both sheep and goat RBC lysed. These are formed by cells making the highly cross-reactive antibody. The remainder would be "partial," the sheep RBC being lysed, but not the goat, producing a localized area of 50% lysis [pictures of such clear and partial plaques can be found in Cunningham, A. J. and Pilarski, L. M. (1974). *Eur. J. Immunol.* **4,** 757].

4.2 By injecting animals with an antigen and then, at various intervals, giving antiserum against the same antigen. This would be found to abort the immune response, particularly if given early. The dose and nature of the serum should be adjusted so as to mimic, as far as possible, the levels of antibody naturally produced during an immune response. The inhibitory powers of different classes of Ig could be distinguished by injecting antibody of only one class into a recipient (ways of separating Ig classes are described in methodology texts, e.g., Ref. 2.7).

4.3 The popliteal node receives lymph only from tissue fluids and not from any more peripheral node: thus most of the cells in its efferent lymph come from the blood. The rate of recirculation of lymphocytes from blood to lymph increases after antigenic stimulation. In addition, large blast cells and basophilic mononuclear cells which are not normally common, appear in efferent lymph of the stimulated node. These cells, many of which make specific antibody, are produced within the node by division from blood-borne small lymphocyte precursors. This can be demonstrated by infusing a DNA label such as ^{3}H-thymidine into the node (via an afferent lymphatic vessel): virtually all of the new morphological cell types take up this label as can be shown by autoradiography of a smear of efferent lymph cells. This topic is discussed further in Hall, J. G. and Morris, B. (1965). *J. Exp. Med.* **121**, 901, and Cunningham, A. J., Smith, J. B., and Mercer, E. H. (1966). *J. Exp. Med.*, **124**, 701.

CHAPTER 5

5.1   Since there are many antigenic differences between *all* cells of two such unrelated species as rabbit and mouse, a rabbit-anti-mouse-thymus cell serum would contain antibodies to many components as well as the θ antigen. It would, therefore, react with all cells in mouse spleen, although possibly to highest titer against T cells. To make such a serum specific, one would like to absorb out (Section 2.1) all anti-mouse antibodies except anti-θ. This is a tricky practical problem, both because of the difficulty of finding populations of mouse lymphoid containing all antigens except θ (i.e., with no T cells) to use as absorbents, and because the rabbit antibody to mouse θ antigen may cross-react with other antigens and be absorbed out by them. As a first step, the serum could be absorbed with mouse erythrocytes, to remove the bulk of irrelevant anti-mouse antibodies. A subsequent absorption with fetal liver might be tried, or with bone marrow (which does, however, contain small numbers of θ-bearing cells). The preparation of such sera is an empirical process; each is different. Absorption would be continued until the serum proved sufficiently selective for its intended use, e.g., to remove helper activity but not B cell activity from a primed cell population.

5.2   The cells could be treated with proteolytic enzymes, under conditions sufficiently mild to strip off projecting proteins without killing the cells. After some hours in culture, new Ig molecules would appear on the surface of cells actively synthesizing such Ig. A more technically difficult (although conceptually elegant) approach to this problem would be to take cells from an individual heterozygous for the allotype (Section 3.3) of cytophilic Ig. Cells making their own Ig would have only one allotype (see also Section 8.1); those absorbing it passively from the serum would have both allotypes, as might be demonstrated by simultaneous staining with two anti-allotype sera, each with a different attached label (e.g., different-colored fluorescent dyes).

5.3   The primary injection of XY induces anti-Y helper T cells which assist the subsequent response by B cells against Z when antigen YZ is administered. This could be verified in a cell transfer experiment: cells from the XY-primed individual should reproduce their strong, rapid response to Z when injected into an irradiated host and challenged with antigen YZ. If, however, the cells are first pretreated with anti-θ serum plus complement to kill the (immune) T cells, and a source of normal T cells is added, the population as a whole would now make only a primary type of adoptive immune response to Z (Section 5.4.3).

CHAPTER 6

6.1   If the initial dose of antigen is very high, cells with high affinity receptors do not have much selective advantage over those with receptors of lower affinity for the antigen: there is enough antigen to stimulate both categories, and affinity of serum antibody matures slowly. By contrast, when very small amounts of antigen are injected, only cells with high affinity can "trap" it and be stimulated to produce serum antibody, whose affinity therefore increases rapidly (Section 6.6).

   While there is undoubtedly some truth in the above conventional explanation of these events, antibody affinity patterns show some anomalies which suggest that, as well as selecting high affinity cells, antigenic stimulation also *creates* these as variants from precursors with lower affinity receptors. (See Section 8.3.5 and Ref. 8.4 for an introduction to this radical literature.)

6.2   The second antigen has a new determinant, Z, to which T cells are not tolerant. Anti-Z T cells might therefore help the response of B cells to all three determinants X, Y, and Z.

This kind of effect has been observed experimentally. Tolerance to one antigen, e.g., a serum albumin may often be broken by injecting a cross-reacting antigen (a different albumin). However, the above explanation, while useful as a framework for understanding the immunological events, is certainly an oversimplification of what really happens (as with probably all scientific hypotheses). Anomalies sometimes appear, which can not be accounted for by the simple scheme, e.g., "antigen XYZ" may induce "anti-W" antibody.

6.3   The proportion of B cells specific for the antigen (sheep erythrocytes) had been increased ten times or more by the preimmunization of the donor mouse. As a result, many more clones of plaque forming cells against this antigen developed on culture.

CHAPTER 7

7.1   As discussed in Section 7.2, the main arguments for somatic mutation are: relatively few genes need to be inherited in the germline, which avoids the problem of losing genes by "genetic drift" and is consistent with recent findings using molecular hybridization; the inheritance of V region allotypes and species-specific residues is more easily explained; it is clear how the individual responds to "unexpected" stimuli. The germline theory, on the other hand, requires no novel mechanism for variation at V gene loci, and it simply explains the subgroup patterns of V region sequences as another example of the evolutionary divergence of genes, which is already well known to occur in other proteins (e.g., cytochromes).

7.2   It would seem to be very difficult to explain self-tolerance on an instructive theory (probably one of the considerations which led Jerne and Burnet back to selectionist ideas). If there were only one kind of immunocompetent cell, making a basic, unfolded, antibody polypeptide, and if this chain simply molded itself around any antigen that got into the cell, then it is hard to see why all such cells would not become committed to making specific antibody against the self-components which surround them.

7.3   No. There could conceivably be equal rates of mutation in V and C genes, but only V region mutants would be selected, antibody receptors with C region changes having no relevance to antigen binding and therefore no selective advantage.

CHAPTER 8

8.1   1 in 256 [i.e., $(\frac{1}{4})^4$, if my arithmetic is correct!]. It seems not unreasonable that most antibodies, chosen at random, would bind to at least one of the many self-components with significant affinity. If only 1 in 10 antibodies remains unaffected by self-antigens the proportion of cells "wasted" (by tolerization) becomes, obviously, much higher still. If each cell has only one receptor, this exponential effect is obviated.

8.2   The upper limit, for the germline theory, is set by the total number of V genes in the DNA of the zygote. At most, $10^3 V_L$ plus $10^3 V_H$ genes could generate 10^6 different antibody combining sites. The total diversity of the species would be very little greater than that of an individual.

If the somatic mutation theory is correct, the question has no exact answer. The number of different antibodies an individual makes depends on how much mutation occurs in his lymphocytes, which in turn depends mainly on the extent and variety of antigenic stimulation he experiences. Since the antibodies made by different individuals, even against the same antigens, will differ widely, the total range of antibodies produced by a species is many orders of magnitude greater than that made by any one individual. Some upper limit would be set by the number of possible combinations of amino acid sequences that can form a combining site.

8.3   The mouse should survive, since as the lymphoid cells of X and Y genetic type mature, they "learn to tolerate" one another. Although we do not yet understand the exact mechanism of mutual tolerance acquired by cells in such irradiation chimeras, it seems likely to be the same as the normal mechanism for developing tolerance to self-antigens.

CHAPTER 9

9.1   "Thymectomized, irradiated, bone marrow-restored mice" (a common experimental tool of the immunologist!) have few mature T cells. They do possess precursor cells which, however, need to spend some days inside a thymus to mature. A nude mouse is similar in many ways: it has normal B cells and precursor cells, and if successfully implanted with a thymus, will develop mature T cells which can reject foreign grafts.

9.2   First, they may act to suppress specifically the original immune response (experimental examples of this are known). Second, they may provoke further antibodies directed against their own idiotypes, i.e., anti-(anti-idiotypes)! This process might continue indefinitely and act as a mechanism of immune regulation (this idea forms the basis of the "network" hypothesis discussed in Section 11.2.2).

9.3   According to our present ideas and ways of explaining immune events, a low or absent anti-X response in X-tolerant mice injected with XY could be caused either by (a) lack of anti-X B cells, or (b) active suppression against the X part of the antigen. If (a) were true, injecting XY should give a normal anti-Y response. In case (b), the anti-Y response should be diminshed relative to controls (see Section 11.2.1, for examples).

9.4   Contact between the mycobacterial antigens and specifically sensitized T cells liberates lymphokines which are nonspecific, i.e., these activate macrophages which will now help to protect the animal against any other intracellular parasite, such as *Listeria*. [For further discussion see Blanden *et al. In* "Immunology of the Macrophage" (D. S. Nelson, ed.), p. 367. Academic Press, New York, 1976.]

CHAPTER 10

10.1   Brothers and sisters have one-half of their genes in common and must therefore share at least 50% of their histocompatibility antigens (their similarity can be greater than this depending on what genes the mother and father had in common). The chances of a sibling graft being accepted is therefore better, on average, than for a graft from a genetically unrelated donor. Grandparents would have only 25% of their DNA in common with the patient, and therefore are less suitable. (They would also provide a rather old kidney!)

10.2   This kidney would pick up AB-type blood lymphocytes from its new host which, on return of the organ to the AA donor, would be attacked by AA lymphocytes, probably causing rejection of the kidney (this has been demonstrated experimentally).

10.3   Box (1) = AB, (2) = AA, and (3) = BC. AA kills AB because the recipient sees no foreign antigens on AA and cannot react against the invading lymphocytes. On the other hand, AA cells react against BC, but are eventually destroyed by the host since A antigens are foreign, etc.

CHAPTER 11

11.1   Clearly, proteins A and B are very similar, but not chemically identical, while protein C is antigenically and, therefore, structurally less closely related. Table 11.1 lists some of the reasons for the unpredictability of immune responses; it is almost always found that different individuals make antisera with different cross-reactivity patterns, like those shown in the table. Each serum is a unique mixture of antibodies with different primary structures. Probably the most important factors contributing to variation between individuals are: differences in prior antigenic history, and chance events in immune induction. Rabbit 4 may have been previously exposed to some environmental antigen which cross-reacts more with B than with A; or the lymphocyte population of rabbit 4 may have developed (by somatic mutation?) a number of immunocompetent cells with receptors of higher affinity for B than for A. If the rabbits came from an outbred colony, they would probably have a different complement of Ir genes (Section 11.3) which would certainly also influence their immune responses (however, the same kinds of variation are seen between genetically identical animals injected with the same antigen).

11.2   As we discussed in Chapter 1, the degree of specificity which the immune system must display is determined by the need to distinguish between self and foreign antigens. If many cells are stimulated by one antigen, some must react against self-components and therefore have to be controlled. The need for *specificity* remains; how this is achieved would not be explained by simply demonstrating suppression of anti-self reactions. This problem, making a highly specific reaction with cells whose individual combinations with antigen are often not very specific, has barely been considered by immunologists. Part of the answer may lie in the dynamic, evolutionary character of lymphocyte responses: cells with low avidity for the antigen are initially stimulated, but do not compete successfully with higher avidity cells; lymphocytes which become stimulated by foreign antigens, but have high avidity for a self-component, may be most liable to regulation by an already existing suppressor mechanism. Several different "levels" of regulation may exist, each with relatively low specificity, but in combination forming a barrier to clonal proliferation through which emerge only those immunologically active cells which have a combination of high avidity for the foreign antigen and low reactivity toward all self-components.

CHAPTER 12

12.1   He has immediate hypersensitivity to antigens associated with mice, probably their skin and hair; that is, he has developed circulating and mast cell-bound IgE antibody specific for these antigens. When inhaled, the mouse antigens combine with the IgE antibody on the surface of mast cells in or near the respiratory tract. The subsequent release, from mast cell granules, of histamine and other vasoactive amines causes constriction of bronchiolar smooth muscle and difficulty in breathing (Section 12.2.3). Mouse antigens rubbed into a scratch on the author's skin provoke a rapid local reddening and swelling which peaks in unpleasantness about 30 minutes later. A bite causes quite extensive local swelling, presumably because of histamine-induced vasodilation.

12.2   It is currently thought that T cells reacting against the new, virus-specified antigens may "help" a response, on the part of B cells or other T cells, against antigens intrinsic to muscle. (If immunocompetent thymus-derived cells are infected by virus, various interesting autoimmune effects are conceivable, as discussed by Bretscher in Ref. 12.2.)

CHAPTER 13

13.1   Immunize some animals with one species of the bacteria, other animals with the other species;

show that washed macrophages only rapidly phagocytize those bacteria against which the animal donating the cells was immunized.

13.2   Examine the sera of cows for specific antibody: if the infection is recent and spreading, periodic samples will show an increasing proportion of positives, and a number of individuals in which serum titers rise with time.

13.3   Because of the phenomenon of "original antigenic sin" explained in Section 13.3.1, the response of the previously immunized person may be diverted into antibody production against the original strain of virus, rather than against the new strain.

CHAPTER 14

14.1   Most tumors transplanted into animals genetically different from the original host are rejected because of the reaction against foreign histocompatibility antigens. If two chemically induced tumors have separate origins, they are likely also to have different tumor-associated transplantation antigens (Section 14.3.2). Antisera able to distinguish the two could be prepared in animals syngeneic with the tumor-bearing individual.

14.2   It seems probable that antibody can clump molecules of antigen into a matrix able to combine multivalently with receptors on the surface of specific immunocompetent cells. As we have discussed in Section 2.3.3 and on several subsequent occasions, multipoint attachments have much higher avidity than combinations between single antigen and antibody molecules. (Such aggregates may also have several free antibody valencies which makes them potentially effective agents for "blanketing" antigens on the tumor itself, preventing access to cytotoxic T cells.) When a primary tumor is removed, antigen is no longer being shed into the serum so its concentration falls: antibody is now in excess (Section 2.2.3) and can prevent matrix formation.

14.3   There is no doubt that immune mechanisms are often important in controlling tumors bearing foreign antigens, such as virus-induced tumors. To this extent there is little difference between the immune surveillance theory and the idea that the immune system has evolved to combat infectious agents. If it were demonstrated that all tumors are caused by extrinsic agents, this would remove one of the current objections to the surveillance theory: that the incidence of "spontaneous" tumors does not increase in immunodeficient animals (Table 14.1). However, as explained in Section 14.4, the surveillance theory also maintains that there is some kind of reciprocal relationship between immune receptors and histocompatibility alloantigens—that a high intrinsic rate of variation in these antigens is important to induce a large number of cells ready to react against tumors whose antigens will "look like" alloantigens; hence, the vigor of allograft reactions. This aspect of the immune surveillance theory seems open to criticism (Section 14.4).

When the dust passes, thou wilt see whether thou ridest a horse or an ass.

                                                                                Oriental Proverb

Index

DATE DUE

DATE DUE			
APR 7 1983			
OCT 0 6 1984			
NOV 1 9 1985			
DEC 1 7 1986			
JAN 2 9 1987			
DEC 2 0 1987			
JAN 2 9 1988			
DEC 2 0 1988			

DEMCO 38-297